ONE DISEASE:
REDOX IMBALANCE

How Stress Becomes Disease

Michael R Sherer

Copyright © 2021 by Michael Sherer

One Disease Redox Imbalance

All rights reserved. No part of this publication may be reproduced, distributed, or transmitted in any form or by any means, including photocopying, recording, or other electronic or mechanical methods, without the prior written permission of the publisher, except in the case of brief quotations embodied in critical reviews and certain other noncommercial uses permitted by copyright law.

Although the author and publisher have made every effort to ensure that the information in this book was correct at press time, the author and publisher do not assume and hereby disclaim any liability to any party for any loss, damage, or disruption caused by errors or omissions, whether such errors or omissions result from negligence, accident, or any other cause.

Adherence to all applicable laws and regulations, including international, federal, state, and local governing professional licensing, business practices, advertising, and all other aspects of doing business in the US, Canada, or any other jurisdiction, is the sole responsibility of the reader and consumer.

Neither the author nor the publisher assumes any responsibility or liability whatsoever on behalf of the consumer or reader of this material. Any perceived slight of any individual or organization is purely unintentional.

The resources in this book are provided for informational purposes only and should not be used to replace the specialized training and professional judgment of a health care or mental health care professional.

Neither the author nor the publisher can be held responsible for the use of the information provided within this book. Please always consult a trained professional before making any decision regarding treatment of yourself or others.

ISBN: 978-1-954234-01-7

Contents

Preface 3

Chapter 1 13
Redox Imbalance, the Emergence of a New Disease 13

Chapter 2 21
The Journey from Free Radicals to Redox Imbalance 21

Chapter 3 31
Quercetin: An Object Lesson in Epistemology 31

Chapter 4 43
Redox Imbalance: The Disease We Don't Treat 43

Chapter 5 67
Redox Imbalance and the Case for Other Root Causes 67
  Root Cause Candidate 1: Genetics/Epigenetics
  and Anti-Aging Research 68
  Root Cause Candidate 2: The Microbiome 71
  The Microbiome: Key Takeaways 73
  Root Cause Candidate 3: NAD+ 74
  Root Cause Candidate 4: Magnesium 76
  Root Cause Candidate 5: Inflammation 78

Chapter 6 81
Diagnosing Redox Imbalance 81
Biomarkers For Oxidative Stress 82
Biomarkers for Reductive Stress 103
Redox Health Biomarkers for Patients 104
Redox Biomarkers: Future Directions 105

Chapter 7 109
Redox Self-care: Prevention Through Resilience 109
Self-care and Resilience Habits 110
Core Resilience Habit #1: Sleep 112
Core Resilience Habit #2: Regular Exercise 118
Core Resilience Habit #3: A Nutrient-dense Diet 129
Resilience Habit: Stay Hydrated 134
Resilience Habit: Calorie Restriction 135
Resilience Habit: Intermittent Fasting 136
Resilience Habit: Mindfulness/Vagus Nerve Stimulation 138
Resilience Habit: Acute Heat Stress 140
Resilience Habit: Acute Cold Stress 141
Resilience Habit: Controlled Hypoxia 141
Resilience Habit: Regular Blood Donation 142
Resilience Habit: Micro-habits 143
Measuring Resilience 145
Resilience Habits: Wrapping Up 146

Chapter 8 149
Treating Redox Imbalance 149
The Science Behind Emerging Redox Health Therapies 153
Reimagining the Doctor–Patient Relationship 159
Exploring the Genome and Exposome Together 160
A Conversation about Resilience Habits 166
A Conversation about Nutrition 168
A Conversation about Aging 185
A Conversation about Prescription Drugs, Over-the-Counter Meds, and Supplements 187
A Conversation about Genetics, Epigenetics, and Signaling 200
A Conversation about Symptoms and Pathologies 207

Therapeutic Goals and Strategies and
Other Disease-Specific Discussions 210
Treating Redox Imbalance: Summing Up 210

Chapter 9 213
Moving Forward, Claiming the Benefits 213
Living Out Redox Health Principles on a Personal Level 214
Thinking Bigger 216
Thinking Ahead 219

Postscript 225
Chasing Health: Reflections on the Journey 225

Appendix A: Redox Glossary 237

If you're reading this, I know you're serious about improving your health. Since hitting the publish button, I've continued to find exciting new health research, resilience tips, recipes, anti-aging strategies and more, and I want to share them with you. I've made it easy: just head to

https://redoxhealth.org/bonus

to sign-up for your bonus content and start your redox health journey. Thank you for your interest and support!

Sincerely,

Michael R Sherer
Author, *One Disease: Redox Imbalance*

One Disease: Redox Imbalance
How Stress Becomes Disease

Preface

Anyone who has perused the health section at a local bookseller has surely noticed this pattern: the author/celebrity/MD identifies a one-sentence thesis that will resonate with some fairly broad population and then spends the next 100 to 300 pages explaining why this thesis will deliver some worthwhile outcome for the reader—a flat belly, lost weight, lowered risk for heart disease or cancer, reversal of diabetes. Here's mine:

"Stress causes disease. Redox imbalance is why."

Intuitively, most people know that stress causes disease. How many times have you heard or even said, "I got this cold because things are really stressful at work and I'm feeling run down"? Or perhaps you've known someone who got hives, cancer, or shingles, had a heart attack, or even died while under stress, and figured there was probably a connection. That said, unless you are a medical researcher, most people have little idea of why stress causes disease.

Over the past decade, an avalanche of scientific papers has been published, building a case for the idea that redox[1] imbalance—typically elevated oxidative stress/diminished antioxidant capacity caused by stress of all kinds—causes disease. The emerging picture is one far more complex than the earlier, simple-but-wrongheaded notion that oxidants are

---

[1] Redox is a shortening of Reduction and Oxidation reactions

bad and antioxidants are good. Rather, the research showed that:

1. Oxidants were essential to healthy signaling and proper function of all bodily systems.
2. Low-level stressors, such as exercise, eating plants, calorie restriction, sunlight, gravity, and cold showers, triggered adaptive responses that made the body more resilient to future stress.
3. The healthy body needed redox (oxidation/reduction) processes to be tightly regulated and had systems to accomplish this while allowing the body to adapt quickly and effectively to its changing environment.
4. Under chronic or extreme stress, these systems could be overwhelmed, resulting in damage, pathological signaling, and dysregulation, ultimately resulting in symptoms and disease.

The idea that the root cause of disease has been hiding in plain sight makes this book part health literature and part mystery novel. How can it be that over 250,000 articles describe the health impacts of oxidative stress on PubMed (a searchable database of peer-reviewed medical research) yet most people have never read or heard anything about it? How can it be that scientists already broadly recognize that oxidative stress and redox imbalance play a leading role in cancer, heart disease, diabetes, aging, depression, dementia, and virtually every other disease in humans, animals, and even plants, but my doctor has never mentioned anything about it?

I became borderline obsessed with solving this mystery—and the book before you is the result, a book more than ten years in the making. In my former role as an IT professional, it was my job to spot trends early and position my organization to take advantage of them. Family health issues turned me into a medical researcher, and about ten years ago I began to notice an increasing number of articles on PubMed on oxidative stress—that it caused or was a significant contributor to heart disease, hypertension, stroke, cancer, diabetes, lung disease, kidney and liver disease, and psoriasis. Oxidative stress was an accelerating trend in health research.

At this point, my efforts shifted to synthesizing a broad range of research to understand how oxidative stress causes disease and why this growing body of research was largely unknown outside of the scientific community. My conclusion was that the insights growing out of this research actually represent a radically different way of thinking about health and disease—a new paradigm that didn't fit the current pharmaceutical and procedure-driven medical system.

I wish this story had a nice straight path to publishing this book and changing the world, but there was a problem. I was an IT professional, not a redox biologist, so although I was reading thousands of articles and gaining a broad understanding of the field, I was not privy to the professional conversations about what the canonical articles were, who the thought leaders were, what the latest developments were, what landmines to avoid and what buttons not to push. Late in the manuscript process, two significant things happened. First, I joined the Society for Redox Biology and Medicine (SfRBM). This organization is home to luminaries in the field, such as Helmut Sies (the father of oxidative stress) and Dean Jones, and scores of up-and-coming researchers doing cutting-edge work to translate concepts from redox biology into clinical medicine. While I still have much to learn from this community, it has already helped me better understand where my earlier work was falling short. Second, in November 2020, Helmut Sies published "Oxidative Stress: Eustress and Distress," a capstone effort for Sies, now 78 years old. At 829 pages, the book stands as a landmark work for the field that reflects on its history, synthesizes the current state of the science and looks to its future. If writing this book was like taking the final exam, reading Sies' book was like looking at the answer key.

These two developments simultaneously provided me with the mandate to raise my game and the touchstone to understand where I was falling short and what needed to be strengthened. So I set to work, absorbing the latest information and reflecting on how it validated or critiqued my own work. The result, I believe, is a stronger book, but in no way a derivative work. My goals are different from Sies' goals or those of SfRBM. I am approaching a body of new research that has demonstrably not crossed over to clinical medicine, but not as a redox biologist or a doctor, but a health consumer, a futurist, an organizational leader, and a strategic planner. I wanted to understand the ramifications of this research—what is known and where the gaps are, where it's headed, what the barriers to acceptance are, and what is actionable now.

Do I still think redox researchers are showing us a different paradigm for understanding health and disease? Absolutely. Western medicine does not currently accept that redox imbalance is a root cause of disease; many researchers clearly do, even if the gaps in knowledge and other epistemological, methodological, and regulatory barriers prevent its application to clinical medicine. I have chosen to frame redox imbalance as a disease, which though provocative, makes a lot of sense. I have allowed myself to imagine a world where we measure, diagnose and treat redox imbalance, and I believe the ramifications of doing so are profound.

Some people will disagree with my opinions, and that's okay. Together we can reach a higher truth. The point is to start a conversation about ideas that could transform healthcare, not a food fight. With 50+ new studies being published daily on the topic, existing knowledge gaps continue to be filled, inferences and predictions will be proven or disproven. If necessary, the model will need to be adjusted to reflect the latest understandings. That's not a problem. That's how science works.

Do I think redox imbalance could be embraced by US healthcare? That's a qualified yes. It can certainly inform how we think about health and disease now. There are already redox therapies available; they simply are not acknowledged and labeled as such. How the industry and regulatory bodies think about evidence, what acceptable therapies are, and who can provide them will determine the role redox therapies play and how long they take to arrive at your doctor's office.

Summing up: this book is not attempting to be a peer-reviewed scientific paper or doctoral thesis, but rather an exploration of the growing body of redox research and its potential ramifications for how we think about health and disease. I've tried to hew closely to the current research, but I reserve the right to summarize or omit things that I think are too far down in the weeds in the interest of brevity and simplicity. I occasionally use terms that may be slightly different from the technical terms, and where I deviate, I'll try to note both that I am doing so and why. Now, on to a brief introduction to the redox health paradigm.

The core of the redox health paradigm is contained in the earlier thesis statement, "Stress causes disease. Redox imbalance is why." That said, I've found it useful to attempt to frame this material in several different lengths and forms—the four hundred-word synopsis, the eighteen-minute TED-style talk, ninety-five theses, an infographic, the consumer-focused book. Each approach has its own special challenges and yields additional insights. For example, in the four hundred-word synopsis presented below, I'm obligated to abstract the details into very high-level, understandable concepts because there's no room to explain the complexities. This is probably the furthest I get from the scientific terminology even while attempting to stay aligned with the underlying principles.

Redox Imbalance: How Stress Causes, Cures, and Prevents Disease (a 400-word synopsis)

Redox Imbalance can be thought of as a progression through three levels: The first being stress, the second being the stress response which restores homeostasis, establishes an adaptation that is different from the original state, or advances to the third level, damage and dysregulation of cells, tissues, and bodily systems.

Level 1: Stress

There are eight categories of stress:

- Psychological (what we typically think of as stress)
- Pathogenic (fungal, bacterial, viral, parasitic infections)
- Toxic (poisons, pharmaceuticals, xenobiotics, heavy metals, biological waste products)
- Nutritional (processed carbohydrates, sugar, trans fats, overconsumption of omega-6 fatty acids, high-heat cooking, allergens, anti-nutrients, overeating, malnourishment)
- Physical (injury, damage, imbalance, physical stress, shear stress, under-use, inactivity)
- Environmental (light, sound, radiation, electromagnetic fields, heat, cold, barometric pressure changes)
- Genetic/epigenetic (genetic variants that affect redox status, DNA damage and mutation, pathological gene expression, and signaling)
- Systemic (damage and dysregulation of your bodily systems)

Level 2: Stress Response

These stressors cause a universal stress response in your cells: overproduction of reactive oxygen, nitrogen, and/or sulfur species (which are toxic but also important foundational signaling molecules that activate protective/defense systems such as the immune system, the sympathetic nervous system, and the endocrine system).

A healthy redox system is stress-resilient, can protect the body from most day-to-day threats, and actually benefits from low levels of oxidative stress, a process known as hormesis. But when stress is too great or prolonged, the redox system can get overwhelmed and dysregulated, resulting in lowered stress resilience, oxidative damage, and pathological signaling.

Level 3: Damage and Dysregulation

Low stress resilience makes you vulnerable to self-sustaining oxidative stress states, inflammatory cascades, and feedforward loops, which are manifested in nine foundational dysregulations that result in disease progression and symptoms in multiple bodily systems.

- Nutritional dysregulation
- Immune dysregulation
- Autonomic dysregulation
- Signaling dysregulation (redox, endocrine, paracrine signaling)
- Microbiome dysregulation
- Metabolic dysregulation
- Genetic/epigenetic dysregulation
- Detoxification dysregulation (liver, kidney, gallbladder, spleen, lymphatic system, etc.)
- Endothelial dysregulation (circulatory system, gut barrier, blood-brain barrier, gut-vascular barrier)

Treating Redox Imbalance

Treatments for redox imbalance would intervene in ways that bolster antioxidant capacity and reduce oxidative stress, addressing oxidative damage and dysregulated signaling so that the body's own healing capacity can restore your health.

Intervention steps:
- Level 1: Identify and mitigate unhealthy stressors.
- Level 2: Bolster and maintain stress resilience with regular exercise, seven to eight hours of high-quality sleep nightly, a nutrient-dense diet, effective stress management, and intelligent supplementation as needed to restore and maintain stress resilience, energy production, and healthy immune function.

- Level 3: Identify and disrupt self-sustaining oxidative stress/inflammatory loops and pro-oxidant states by addressing nutritional deficits, pathogenic sources, and biochemical imbalances; pharmaceuticals and surgery are a last resort.

The 400-word synopsis gives additional information but raises plenty of its own questions: Where do these ideas come from? What does dysregulation really mean? What's the difference between stress and oxidative stress? How does redox imbalance cause individual diseases? And so, at the end of it all, the 200-page book is still necessary—to explain, to explore, to convince, to inspire change.

The Simplicity of the Idea. The Complexity of the Science

People ask me, "Who is this book for?" and I've struggled with that question because although I've worked hard to make the material accessible, I've also tried to make it reflect the latest scientific research, which is complex. The book is grounded in the belief that ordinary people, with some guidance, can read and benefit from reading primary scientific research. I've known patients who have been so highly motivated to understand their conditions that they far surpass their doctors in specific knowledge. I've known others who have put incurable diseases into remission and significantly improved their quality of life through experimentation and discipline.

So in the end, this book is for anyone who has wondered whether the current medical paradigm, with its high costs and focus on pills and procedures, is the only or even the best evidence-based approach to health, or for anyone who has been told their condition has no known cause and/or no cure, or anyone who has been told they have multiple autoimmune conditions, or anyone whose medications are causing health issues as concerning as the original condition, or anyone who believes that the cost of the current healthcare system is unsustainable for even the wealthiest country in the world.

The Silent Pandemic: Redox Imbalance and COVID-19

At the time of this writing, the world is in the midst of the COVID-19 pandemic—an oxidative stress-driven disease[2,3] that kills the sick and the aged. Beyond killing nearly three million globally and over 500,000 in the US, the pandemic has exposed a critical weakness in our existing approach to health and disease—to the extent that it treats symptoms rather than root causes, it manages rather than cures chronic disease. In so doing, we've created a society where six in 10 adults have one or more chronic diseases and are thus more vulnerable to getting COVID cases severe enough to hospitalize or kill them. Worse yet, by ignoring the root causes of disease and the strategies that build resilience, we continue down our path to societal ill health, chronic disease, and vulnerability to the next pandemic.

It doesn't have to be this way. Through advances in redox biology, genetics, epigenetics, nutrition, and -omics fields, science shows us a better path that we can benefit from today. This book is about those advances. If it in any way helps the people who read it move in the direction of better health and greater resilience to stressors of all kinds, every effort in writing it, in sweating the details, in integrating disparate fields, in getting it as close to right as current science allows, will have been worth it.

Michael Sherer

Standard disclaimer: I am not a doctor; this book is not medical advice.

---

2 Suhail, Shanzay et al. "Role of Oxidative Stress on SARS-CoV (SARS) and SARS-CoV-2 (COVID-19) Infection: A Review." *The protein journal* vol. 39,6 (2020): 644-656. doi:10.1007/s10930-020-09935-8

3 Beltrán-García, Jesús et al. "Oxidative Stress and Inflammation in COVID-19-Associated Sepsis: The Potential Role of Anti-Oxidant Therapy in Avoiding Disease Progression." *Antioxidants (Basel, Switzerland)* vol. 9,10 936. 29 Sep. 2020, doi:10.3390/antiox9100936

Dedicated to Lon Sherer (1932–2018)
Father, friend, and fellow experimenter

Many thanks to:
- Helmut Sies, Dean Jones, and the many redox biology researchers for your vision and tenacity in bringing oxidative stress and redox imbalance into the scientific mainstream.
- Dr. Joel Fuhrman, T. Colin Campbell, Caldwell Esselstyn, Dean Ornish and others who put me onto the life-saving benefits of plant-based, nutrient-dense eating.
- Margie Davis, RN, John Martens, MD, Jonathan Neufeld, Ph.D., Patsy Sherer, Duane Stoltzfus, Ph.D., and others for their invaluable feedback on the manuscript as it went through many rewrites.
- Ray Sylvester for being a great editor. You truly did make this a better book in so many ways.

Chapter 1

Redox Imbalance, the Emergence of a New Disease

> "He who cures a disease may be the skillfullest, but he that prevents it is the safest physician."
> — Thomas Fuller, 17th-century author

Once every few years, a new disease appears that captures the public imagination—HIV, Legionnaires' disease, SARS, avian influenza, Ebola, Zika, and most recently, COVID-19. The specter of the disease running rampant through society mobilizes the media, public health community, governmental structures, and the medical industry. Articles explaining the disease and its threat are written. Strategies for controlling the outbreak are devised. The search for vaccines and effective treatment commences. Federal dollars for research are reallocated. Foundations to raise funds for its eradication are created. Progress (or lack of it) is chronicled in the media.

Now imagine a new disease so serious that it has the potential to kill everyone on the planet, so pervasive that everyone gets it, so costly that it drives over a trillion dollars of healthcare spending annually in the US alone, so foundational that it is a root cause of all chronic disease, and so disruptive that it has the potential to change how we think about health and disease, how we do medical research, and how we deliver healthcare. This book is about that disease—what it is, the scientific foundation for it, and paradoxically, why most people have never heard of it.

That disease is redox imbalance. Although you will most likely die from redox imbalance and its downstream effects, there are no foundations calling for its eradication (yet), no drumbeat of daily health articles describing our progress in controlling or eradicating it. Your doctor has never tested you for it, diagnosed it, or treated it. Yet it is behind all of the Center for Disease Control's (CDC) top twelve causes of death except, arguably, accidental death.

The idea that something so important and so foundational could be hiding in plain sight is almost unbelievable. Yet as I sought answers to family health challenges on PubMed, a global database of health research, the concepts of oxidative stress, antioxidant capacity, nitrosative stress, oxidative damage, and redox signaling were everywhere. What's more, many scientists were demonstrating and declaring that oxidative stress and loss of antioxidant capacity were central to the onset and progression of cancer, heart disease, diabetes, obesity, lung, kidney, and liver disease, depression, neurodegenerative diseases, and virtually every other chronic disease, as well as the symptoms and pathologies of infectious diseases such as the common cold, flu, HIV and COVID-19.

At the time of this writing, over 250,000 articles on PubMed mention oxidative stress, over 95 percent of them written since 2000, with over a thousand more appearing each month. With each passing month, the picture becomes clearer, and the story becomes more compelling, yet the question remains: Why hasn't this information done more to change healthcare? To answer this, we first need to engage some foundational ideas from epidemiology.

As the name implies, epidemiology arose out of the need to understand and mitigate infectious disease outbreaks—epidemics. Modern epidemiology has become broadly focused on all disease, defined as the study of the incidence, distribution, and control of disease in a population. In *Epidemiology 101,* we learn about the Epidemiologic Triangle, the "Who, What and Where" of disease. In it, the **Host** is the "Who," the entity who gets the disease. The **Agent** is the "What," the cause of the disease and the **Environment** is the "Where," the conditions external to the host that cause the disease or allow it to spread. The epidemiologist's role is to disrupt one or more of the legs of that triangle, thereby preventing the disease or its spread.

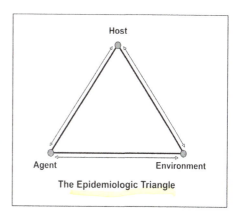

The Epidemiologic Triangle

The COVID-19 pandemic has given the world a crash course in epidemiology that aptly illustrates the epidemiologic triangle. Since the appearance of a mystery respiratory illness in Wuhan, China, in December 2019, we've witnessed the scientific and public health communities' efforts to understand and tackle the emerging pandemic threat and ultimately to disrupt the legs of the epidemiologic triangle. To summarize:

The Agent: SARS-CoV-2 (COVID-19 virus)
- Classification: Coronavirus
- Transmissibility: Highly infectious, a trait compounded by the fact that infected individuals can spread the virus while asymptomatic.
- Pathogenicity: It is significantly higher than seasonal flu, though lower than the original SARS-CoV virus and significantly lower than MERS-CoV. Current estimates of the COVID-19 death rate are approximately 0.5% after asymptomatic cases are factored in.
- Infection process: the virus enters the cell via the ACE2 receptor. The spike glycoprotein binds to the ACE2 receptor, making it a desirable target for vaccines and therapeutic interventions.

The Host: Uninfected humans, with some evidence of transmission to pets and zoo animals from human contact. Susceptibility attributes:
- Sex: Men slightly more susceptible than women.
- Age: Age increases severity and mortality risks.

- Race: Non-whites have experienced increased severity and higher mortality rates.
- Comorbidities/risk factors: Obesity, diabetes, cancer, heart and lung disease, immune deficiencies.
- Complications:
  - Pneumonia and trouble breathing
  - Organ failure in several organs
  - Heart problems
  - A severe lung condition that causes a low amount of oxygen to go through your bloodstream to your organs (acute respiratory distress syndrome)
  - Blood clots
  - Acute kidney injury
  - Additional viral and bacterial infections
  - Post-recovery symptoms

The Environment: Transmission of the virus is primarily through respiratory droplets. Though the virus can survive on surfaces, transmission through touching infected surfaces is considered relatively low risk. Factors favoring transmission:

- Location: Indoor environments. Proper ventilation, filtration, and the introduction of fresh air may reduce transmission.
- Duration: Exposures greater than 15 minutes over 24 hours.
- Proximity: Within 6 feet.

Disruption Strategies: Public Health officials, researchers, and medical professionals have deployed various strategies to disrupt the three legs of the epidemiologic triangle:

Agent-Host:
- Vaccine
- Anti-viral treatments

Environment-Host:
- Social distancing
- Sheltering in place
- Hand-washing for 20 seconds
- Business closures/curfews (e.g., limit access to high-risk locations)

Environment-Agent:
- Self-quarantine of infected persons (e.g., keep infected people away from the uninfected)
- Disinfecting surfaces
- Travel restrictions (e.g., prevent the virus from spreading to unaffected locations)

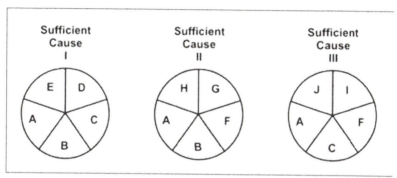

Source: Rothman KJ. Causes. Am J Epidemiol 1976;104:587-592.

While the epidemiologic triangle works well for infectious diseases, it is less satisfactory for chronic diseases, which typically have multiple causes. So while we could attempt to map redox imbalance onto the epidemiologic triangle, it's more helpful to apply a model designed to address multiple-causality. That model is known as "**The Sufficient-Component Cause Model**" or, more colloquially, "Rothman's Pies."[4] Professor Ken Rothman proposed the model in 1976 to provide a more robust theoretical framework for understanding disease causation. In the diagram, each pie represents a "Sufficient Cause," a collection of components that together constitute a complete causal mechanism that will inevitably produce disease. The model recognizes that the individual components that collectively produce disease may differ from case to case, hence the three pies, each with a different set of components represented as slices ranging from A to J.

Oxidative stress/redox imbalance could map onto this causation model in one of three ways:

---
[4] Rothman, K J. "Causes." American journal of epidemiology vol. 104,6 (1976): 587-92. doi:10.1093/oxfordjournals.aje.a112335

1. As a sufficient cause unto itself, meaning that redox imbalance itself is the disease's sole cause.
2. As an insufficient but necessary cause, meaning it will induce the disease only when combined with other components, but it must be present for the disease to occur.
3. As a non-necessary component cause, meaning it can contribute to the disease's onset in some cases. Still, there are other sufficient cause scenarios where the disease occurs, and oxidative stress is not present.[5]

Strictly speaking, if the body's redox systems are truly mediating the adaptive response to internal and external stressors, scenario 1 should never occur. Redox imbalance would only cause disease in combination with other component causes. Similarly, scenario 3 should never occur because the body's redox systems will always be involved in successful and unsuccessful adaptation to stressors—the successful adaptations leading to homeostasis and resilience, and the unsuccessful adaptations leading to symptoms and disease. That would be true even if the redox imbalance is not measurable by existing biomarkers and collection strategies.

Earlier in chapter 1, I raised the idea that a root cause of disease has been hiding in plain sight, and it's a provocative one. But I can think of no better strategy for hiding it than for it to be an insufficient but necessary cause. This is a pretty big deal. Being an insufficient cause diverts your attention to other components that are more visible. Being a necessary cause in every disease allows us to miss it because its very ubiquity makes it blend in, like background noise in an otherwise silent room or gravity. That at least partially explains why we've missed redox imbalance. But the big deal is that if redox imbalance truly is a necessary cause in every disease, then learning to manage redox imbalance and mitigate the stressors that cause it holds the key to treating every disease.

---

5 Ghezzi, Pietro. "Environmental risk factors and their footprints in vivo - A proposal for the classification of oxidative stress biomarkers." *Redox biology* vol. 34 (2020): 101442. doi:10.1016/j.redox.2020.101442

This is where I expect the skeptics to object—"Michael, you can't prove that redox imbalance is a necessary cause in every disease. That would take decades!" To which I would respond, if redox biologists Helmut Sies and Dean Jones are correct (and I think they are) that redox networks form a system that mediates the ability of an organism and its cells to adapt to environmental stress, then it's already true.[6] The experimental validation of that truth will follow, and the relevant systems will behave in ways that support the hypothesis. I've been following this field long enough to say with some confidence that it's already playing out in exactly this way.

That said, to prove redox imbalance is causal in even a single disease, we will need to have a biomarker strategy that supports the hypothesis in a clinical setting. We'll cover biomarkers in greater depth in Chapter 6.

Causality has often been referred to as the holy grail of epidemiology. It has both the elements of a religious quest and an elusive nature that defies iron-clad proof, even in the highest quality studies. The key epidemiological concepts here are **reverse causation** and **confounders**.

In critiques of the oxidative stress theory of disease, numerous authors have observed that both these phenomena could be going on and should give us humility in interpreting the data.[7] For example, if we observe oxidative stress in every case of a disease (e.g., diabetes), we might assume that oxidative stress causes that disease. Still, logically, you could also conclude that diabetes causes oxidative stress—reverse causation. It's also worth pointing out that both causation and reverse causation can occur in complex biological systems, often so rapidly that it's difficult to prove conclusively which came first. When we see this occurring, it's often in the context of something known as a feed-forward loop, or more

---

6 Jones, Dean P, and Helmut Sies. "The Redox Code." *Antioxidants & redox signaling* vol. 23,9 (2015): 734-46. doi:10.1089/ars.2015.6247

7 Ghezzi, Pietro et al. "The oxidative stress theory of disease: levels of evidence and epistemological aspects." British journal of pharmacology vol. 174,12 (2017): 1784-1796. doi:10.1111/bph.13544

colloquially as a vicious cycle, which frequently occurs in disease states. We'll look at this in greater depth in Chapter 4.

Confounders are variables that distort the relationship between a cause and an effect. For example, we might look at the data and assume that A causes C, but in reality, confounder B is causing both A and C. There's an irony that throughout the COVID pandemic, I've been writing this book, all the while thinking oxidative stress/redox imbalance IS the confounder—that causal agent we're overlooking. Healthy redox status confers resilience, so you don't get severe COVID. Aging and comorbid conditions such as diabetes and obesity deplete stress resilience. Respiratory illnesses are massive oxidative stressors. Sepsis and the cytokine storm are major oxidative stress events, and oxidative stress drives the multiple organ failure that leads to COVID death. Oxidative stress and depleted stress resilience even explain the COVID long-hauler symptoms of heart, liver, kidney damage, brain fog, body aches, joint pain, etc. If correct, that opens the tantalizing possibility that we could intervene to help prevent, mitigate, and speed the recovery from COVID-19.

As systems biology progressively reveals the astounding complexity of the systems underlying health and disease, I suspect that Rothman's pies will look increasingly inadequate to explain what's going on. A systems approach will ultimately be necessary to sort out the interrelationships between the myriad causes and effects that ultimately lead to disease. It's a reminder that we're on a journey of discovery—one that should lead to better health and better healthcare.

Chapter 2

The Journey from Free Radicals to Redox Imbalance

> *"Life is nothing but an electron looking for a place to rest."*
> —Nobel Prize-winning physiologist, Albert Szent-Györgyi

Unless you are a biologist or chemist, the word *"redox"* is probably an unfamiliar term to you. Linguistically, it is simply a shortening of the words *reduction* and *oxidation*, which are foundational biochemical processes in both plant and animal cell biology. An oxidation reaction happens when an atom loses an electron to another atom, and a reduction reaction occurs when an atom gains an electron. So a redox reaction is the pairing of an oxidation reaction and a reduction reaction.

Redox reactions, which underlie respiration (breathing) and glucose metabolism (energy production), are foundational to the life and function of every cell in your body and most organisms on the planet. If these redox reactions are not happening inside of you, you are dead. But if they go wrong, they are dangerous.

Oxidative stress, a form of redox imbalance, occurs when the over-production of reactive species outstrips your cells' ability to detoxify them. Medical researchers call this a pro-oxidant state, and when you are in it, you get tissue damage, dysregulated signaling, immune system activation, inflammation, disrupted protein synthesis, cell death, oxidized DNA, oxidized lipids, proteins, and carbohydrates.

Fire is the form of oxidation we are most familiar with, and, as with fire, when your body is in a pro-oxidant state, things get damaged or destroyed. Pushing the fire analogy further, smoke is analogous to redox signaling. Just as too much smoke can be a greater problem than the fire, pathological redox signaling turns out to be a very significant factor in disease initiation and progression. Given enough time, oxidative damage and redox signaling dysregulation will inevitably lead to aging, systemic imbalances, loss of function, disease symptoms, health crises, and ultimately death. Perhaps paradoxically, low levels of oxidative stress have also been recognized as essential to healthy signaling in every cell and bodily system. The scientific exploration of how this all works spans much of the last century, and the underlying physical realities are likely billions of years older.

According to fossil evidence and evolutionary studies, life on earth evolved to utilize oxygen about 3.5 billion years ago in response to what has been termed the "Great Oxygenation Event." According to this theory, cyanobacteria-like organisms developed the ability to use sunlight to extract O_2 from CO_2 and water, and these became the basis for modern-day plant chloroplasts. Over a period of millions of years, the earth's atmosphere became increasingly oxygen-rich—a catastrophe for anaerobic organisms and a boon to organisms that developed systems to detoxify and regulate oxygen in the body. We see evolutionary evidence of these redox regulatory systems in the glutathione, NAD/NADH, and NADP/NADPH systems, as well as evidence of earlier systems able to deal with reactive nitrogen and sulfur species.

Modern-day understandings of oxidative stress/redox imbalance as root causes of disease originate from two different scientific streams, stress research, and free radical biology. The idea that stress causes disease, that there is good and bad stress (eustress and distress), and that stress itself has a very broad definition is not new. It dates back to the 1930s and the pioneering work of Hungarian-Canadian researcher Hans Selye, known as the "father of stress research."

Selye had worked in a clinical setting in the 1920s and noticed that patients with different diseases shared common symptoms. When he shifted into research work, Selye was initially looking for a hormone that caused these symptoms. What he found instead was that multiple kinds of stress produced a common symptomology in his test animals—enlarged adrenal glands, atrophy of the lymphatic system, and peptic ulcers of the stomach and duodenum.[8] Out of this work and subsequent research, Selye formulated his "general adaptation syndrome" (GAS) and introduced the idea of stress into the medical lexicon as the *"nonspecific response of the body to any demand."*

His work both predated and shaped biochemical research underlying modern understandings of the role of stress in disease pathology. It has also shaped popular understandings of stress in mental and physical health (e.g., post-traumatic stress disorder, PTSD). In Selye's GAS model (shown in the figure below), stress resilience in Stage 2: Resistance, would prevent or delay progression to Stage 3: Exhaustion, by facilitating recovery or adaptation. Similarly, loss of stress resilience would both precipitate and be a symptom of Stage 3: Exhaustion, leading to declining health, disease progression, and ultimately death. We will cover stress resilience as a core concept in more detail in the subsequent chapters.

The significance of Selye's work to redox imbalance and oxidative stress is how accurately it predicted the arc of antioxidant defense in the face of an initial stress insult, followed by chronic stress degrading antioxidant capacity until it is exhausted. From today's biochemical perspective, we would describe this as the oxidative stress-driven upregulation of cellular defenses by NRF2 (Stage 1: Alarm), followed by the steady, stress-driven decline of reduced glutathione and other antioxidant systems (Stage 2: Resistance) into a state of redox imbalance that corresponds to Stage 3: Exhaustion. This

---

8 Tan, Siang Yong, and A Yip. "Hans Selye (1907-1982): Founder of the stress theory." Singapore medical journal vol. 59,4 (2018): 170-171. doi:10.11622/smedj.2018043

book is necessarily based on an incomplete understanding of how all these disease mechanisms work. Still, as with Selye's work, I anticipate and have witnessed that the basic paradigm accurately predicts new discoveries. They fill in gaps in our understanding without altering the foundational paradigm.

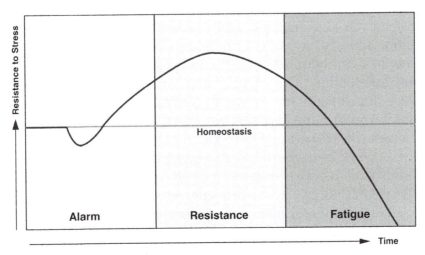

***General Adaptation Syndrome*[9]**
In the 1930s, Hans Selye, "The father of stress research," proposed the general adaptation syndrome (GAS) as a model for understanding the organism's response to stress.

The second stream feeding into modern understandings of redox imbalance comes from free radical biology of the 1950s when Denham Harman postulated the Free Radical Theory of Aging. In his theory, Harman postulated that in all organisms, accumulating damage from free radicals resulted in what we understand to be aging. In the 1970s, Harman extended his theory to include mitochondrial production of reactive oxygen species (ROS), and this work fed into Helmut Sies's coinage of the term oxidative stress in 1985. The free radical theory of aging suggested that therapeutic quenching of free radicals with antioxidants could play a role in preventing disease. Indeed, antioxidant vitamins A, C, E, and beta carotene have

---

[9] David G. Myers, CC BY 3.0, via Wikimedia Commons

been heavily studied, and while they have therapeutic value, they also were no silver bullet. Megadoses of antioxidants did not cure cancer. Sometimes they made it worse.

From Damage to Dysregulation

In recent years, scientific focus has shifted from the damage caused by oxidative stress to the signaling function of redox molecules like hydrogen peroxide (H_2O_2). Your body has a complex signaling network, continuously monitoring its environment and adapting to changes and threats to maintain homeostasis or balance. Scientists have discovered that redox molecules play significant roles in this network, activating:

- The hypothalamic-pituitary-adrenal (HPA) axis (your stress hormone system).
- The sympathetic nervous system (your fight-or-flight system).
- The renin-angiotensin-aldosterone system (to regulate your autonomic nervous system).
- The immune system (to fight a pathogenic stressor or clean up the oxidative damage).
- Cellular defense mechanisms (via the NRF2 pathway)
- Metabolic regulation mechanisms (via the AMPK pathway)
- The Unfolded Protein Response (to prevent and repair misfolded proteins)
- The DNA damage response (to repair both nuclear and mitochondrial DNA damage)
- The hypoxia response to low oxygen situations (via hypoxia-inducible factors)
- The heat/cold shock response to rapid changes in temperature (via heat and cold shock proteins)

Furthermore, redox signaling is involved in gene activation/deactivation, regulation of gene expression, cell differentiation, and cellular functions, including programmed cell death (apoptosis), blood vessel growth (angiogenesis), cell death (necrosis), deterioration (senescence), cellular recycling (autophagy), and cell proliferation (which can lead to cancer). These discoveries have led to burgeoning research interest in oxidative stress and how it impacts health and disease—with 1,000-plus new articles appearing each month.

Redox Compartmentalization

The notion of a pro-oxidant state suggested that oxidative stress could be framed as a systemic condition—over-production of oxidants with too little antioxidant capacity to detoxify them. In the last decade, research into redox signaling again showed this view to be an oversimplification. Redox states varied for different parts of the cell and different redox couples leading to the idea of redox compartments with local protein targets for distinct biological processes.[10]

Reductive Stress: Another Kind of Redox Imbalance

The rising prominence of oxidative stress as a cause of disease inevitably led to attempts to treat it. While there were many successes in this vein, researchers discovered that N-acetylcysteine, which raises your body's glutathione levels, blunted the benefits of exercising! It turns out that low levels of oxidative stress, such as those found in exercise, calorie restriction, ketogenic diets, eating plants, cold stress, and even ionizing radiation, can actually be beneficial, a process known as **hormesis**. Oversupplying the body with antioxidants creates "reductive stress" by driving redox signaling levels below beneficial levels. Reductive stress is less prominent than oxidative stress but can play a role in the development of

---

10 Jones, D P, and Y-M Go. "Redox compartmentalization and cellular stress." Diabetes, obesity & metabolism vol. 12 Suppl 2,Suppl 2 (2010): 116-25. doi:10.1111/j.1463-1326.2010.01266.x

mitochondrial diseases, metabolic syndrome, and conditions like pulmonary hypertension.

The role of reductive stress in metabolic disease is increasingly acknowledged thanks to a deepening understanding of the role of NAD+, an oxidant, in regulating metabolism. Paradoxically, reductive stress in the form of depleted NAD+ results in increased oxidative stress through dysregulated energy production. I liken it to a four-cylinder engine running on three cylinders. If you've experienced such an engine, it runs rough, lacks power and efficiency, and belches out smoke. Similarly, low NAD+ levels result in less energy production and overproduction of reactive oxygen species in the mitochondria, your cells' energy factories, and the result is increased oxidative stress and pathological redox signaling.

Redox Systems, Redox Homeostasis, and the Ability to Adapt

The reality that redox reactions are actually quite dangerous and thus needed to be tightly regulated, led to the elucidation of multiple redox systems with distinct but overlapping functionality. Research into these systems described how they work and their roles in various systems and led to the idea that redox systems were the interface between an organism and its environment.[11] Redox systems could rapidly sense environmental changes (stressors) and via redox signaling, effect useful adaptations that enhanced survival and resilience to future stress. You can think of this as a kind of unconscious biological learning process. The stressor is the lesson, and the adaption is the lesson learned—one that better prepares the organism to handle a similar stressor in the future.

---

11 Go, Young-Mi, and Dean P Jones. "Redox theory of aging: implications for health and disease." Clinical science (London, England : 1979) vol. 131,14 1669-1688. 30 Jun. 2017, doi:10.1042/CS20160897

Beyond Free Radicals and ROS: the Interactome

While early research into redox signaling focused almost entirely on free radical signaling via H_2O_2 and superoxide, scientists increasingly recognized that the complexity of redox signaling implied that a broad palette of reactive species was necessary to deliver that complexity. This realization led to the concept of the reactive species interactome (RSI).[12] The RSI is composed of 22 reactive oxygen, nitrogen, and sulfur species which together allow the organism to sense environmental change and adapt quickly and appropriately. The RSI is a subset of the larger protein-protein interactions network database, consisting of over 100,000 protein interactions.

The Present and Future of Redox Research

At the time of publication, I would summarize the state of redox research as follows:

- Accumulating evidence supports a central role for oxidative stress in aging and a broad range of diseases and disease pathologies.
- Low levels of oxidative stress are typically eustressors that activate the cellular stress response, elicit useful adaptive responses, and improve resilience to future similar stressors.
- Overproduction of oxidants and chronic stress are typically pathological—distress, leading to unregulated oxidation, cellular damage, and pathological signaling.
- Redox signaling and redox regulation of signaling is complex, involving a broad range of reactive oxygen, nitrogen, and sulfur species (the redox interactome) interacting with your body's proteins, lipids,

---

12 Cortese-Krott, Miriam M et al. "The Reactive Species Interactome: Evolutionary Emergence, Biological Significance, and Opportunities for Redox Metabolomics and Personalized Medicine." Antioxidants & redox signaling vol. 27,10 (2017): 684-712. doi:10.1089/ars.2017.7083

carbohydrates, DNA, and RNA to regulate and modulate cell differentiation, genetic expression, cellular defense and adaptation, protein and energy production, the cell life cycle, and various other biological processes. These interactions are being systematically documented.

- Redox status and signaling are highly localized (redox compartments), with local redox-sensitive targets and pathways. The implication here is that oxidation and redox signaling is purposeful and systematic in its physiologic form.
- Oxidative stress can result from multiple paths, internal and external to the body. UV radiation and xenobiotics from skin products affect skin cells directly with systemic effects, particulate air pollution affects lung epithelial cells directly with systemic effects, traffic noise activates the HPA axis and upregulates cortisol with associated oxidative stress, mitochondria produce reactive species as a normal part of energy production, dysregulated mitochondria overproduce reactive species, psychological stressors activate the sympathetic nervous system and, through catecholamine release, activate microglia in the brain with inflammatory neuroimmune effects.
- Oxidative processes are necessary for healthy development, function, and adaptation (eustress). Still, almost all redox processes and signaling have eustress and distress manifestations ranging from too low, to just right, to too high, or too long.
- Despite an increasingly detailed and compelling description of how redox processes are involved in health and disease, there are still almost no acknowledged redox therapies approved and used in clinical practice. At the same time, redox research helps explain how existing therapies work and occasionally, why they don't.

Research into redox health-related issues continues to yield exciting breakthroughs and an ever-deepening understanding of how the body works, how it devolves into disease, and how we might intervene more effectively to maintain and restore health. The impact of all this new information on the actual healthcare you might receive from your doctor or hospital? Frustratingly little. The answer to why lies, I believe, in the esoteric world of epistemology.

Chapter 3

Quercetin: An Object Lesson in Epistemology

> *"Don't believe everything you read on the Internet."*
> *– Abraham Lincoln*

How do we know what is true? How do we separate fact, or at least justified belief, from opinion? What methods and evidence help us evaluate what is valid and likely to work? The discipline of epistemology explores the ins and outs of knowledge and how we know what we know. Just a few years ago, I would have considered a discourse on epistemology to be esoteric to the point of irrelevance. However, in the age of fake news and alternate facts, I'd say we're experiencing an epistemological crisis. Societal agreement on how we evaluate information turns out to be *really* important. It also matters in medicine, but as I studied redox imbalance and reflected on my own experience with western medicine, I began to wonder whether the hierarchy of evidence that undergirds "Evidence-Based Medicine" (EBM) is serving us as well as it needs to in an era of rapidly expanding knowledge of how the body and disease actually work. To understand why and how it affects the non-impact of redox biology on medicine, I offer you the case of the plant polyphenol quercetin:

I have oxidative-stress-driven seasonal allergies. There are months of the year where I was almost non-functional due to the sneezing, runny nose, and watery eyes brought on by high pollen counts or simple tasks like mowing the lawn. Early in my research on oxidative stress, I ran across quercetin, a polyphenol found in apples, onions, and numerous other plants.

According to research, quercetin enhances antioxidant defenses and reduces oxidative stress by stimulating a protein/transcription factor called nuclear factor erythroid 2–related factor 2 or simply NRF2. I noted that it was a natural antihistamine and decided to give it a try. It worked brilliantly. Whenever I felt an allergy attack coming on, two quercetin capsules stopped it, typically within minutes.

Whereas the over-the-counter allergy meds had some potentially worrisome side effects—such as dementia, heart arrhythmias, anxiety, and depression, quercetin seemed to have primarily side benefits. It prevented atherosclerosis in exercising rats, it raised stress resilience, it was anti-diabetic and anti-obesity, killed cancer stem cells, it improved gut flora composition, it helped prevent Alzheimer's disease, it was anti-inflammatory, it prevented anxiety and depression, and offered a host of other health benefits including efficacy in inhibiting COVID-19 infection.[13]

While many of these studies were on rodents or *in vitro*, an increasing number of studies on humans are showing equally impressive results. I take quercetin daily and credit it with dramatically reducing the number of upper respiratory infections I have had over the past decade, an observation with increasing research evidence.[14] This alone has definitely improved my quality of life and probably extended it as well.

Yet despite having access to over 20,000 articles on PubMed, most of them extolling the benefits of quercetin in a broad array of health conditions, your doctor is unlikely to recommend that you take it. The Cochrane medical database has no articles

---

13 Solnier, Julia, and Johannes-Paul Fladerer. "Flavonoids: A complementary approach to conventional therapy of COVID-19?." *Phytochemistry reviews : proceedings of the Phytochemical Society of Europe*, 1-23. 18 Sep. 2020, doi:10.1007/s11101-020-09720-6

14 Somerville, Vaughan S, et all. "Effect of Flavonoids on Upper Respiratory Tract Infections and Immune Function: A Systematic Review and Meta-Analysis." *Advances in Nutrition*, Volume 7, Issue 3, May 2016, Pages 488–497, doi.org/10.3945/an.115.010538

specifically devoted to it. Even my local Walgreens doesn't carry it. If quercetin were a pharmaceutical, there would be studies and newspaper articles guilting doctors into prescribing it and patients into taking it. Newsflash: "Millions of patients with elevated oxidative stress levels are going untreated." There would be heartwarming TV commercials with smiling old people playing with their grandchildren promoting daily quercetin use, followed by incredibly short disclaimers. And, of course, the cost would go from fifteen cents to five dollars a pill, and your insurance company would cover it.

As a natural compound, quercetin isn't patentable, and thus there is no big payday for promoting it and no insurance subsidy for buying it. So, this incredibly useful compound languishes in alternative medicine land, along with many other equally useful natural compounds—polyphenols, minerals, amino acids, vitamins, and herbals. In the name of evidence-based medicine, we are often told that all supplements are ineffective and a waste of money, even when there is abundant evidence to the contrary. I say this even while acknowledging that it is nearly always best to get your nutrients from food.

There are several striking lessons from the case of quercetin:

Levels of Evidence for Certain Benefits are High

You might reasonably assume that quercetin as a non-prescription therapy lacks evidence to warrant its use, but actually, the level of evidence for its efficacy is quite high on multiple fronts. There were 25 systematic reviews and meta-analyses on quercetin at the time of publication, and meta-analyses are at the top of the evidence pyramid. They showed that quercetin:
- Lowers LDL
- Lowers systolic blood pressure
- Lowers fasting glucose
- Reduces the incidence of upper respiratory infections by 33% and lowered sick days by 40%.

- Significantly reduces C-reactive protein levels (a biomarker of inflammation)
- May reduce the risk of colorectal cancer
- May reduce the risk of lung cancer in smokers

So quercetin isn't being ignored because it doesn't work. It's ignored because it's not an FDA-approved pharmaceutical for the above use-cases. The FDA is tasked with protecting consumers from unsafe or unproven medications, so naturally, they discourage consumers from taking unapproved meds. Doctors have legitimate liability concerns, so frankly, why would they take the risk of prescribing a nutritional supplement?

Levels of evidence for other benefits are low, or are they?

WebMD has the following to say about quercetin: "In general, much of the research on quercetin has been in animals or cell cultures. More study is needed to prove quercetin's benefits and safety in humans, especially when taken as a supplement instead of in food."[15] The implication is that the evidence is weak, but is that really accurate? Among those 20,000+ studies on PubMed are, yes, many observational, animal, and cell culture studies that EBM ranks at the bottom of the evidence hierarchy. But something interesting happened in the last two decades that is turning our epistemological world upside down, and it's known in the research world as -omics. For the uninitiated, my short explanation of the -omics craze is that it grew out of the idea that as we sequenced the human genome, we were both creating the need to study a class of newly identified information—genes, and a collection of powerful tools to perform the work. Thus, from genome came genomics, and in the ensuing years, a flood of other -omes and -omics followed:
- Epigenome and epigenomics—the body of epigenetic modifications and the study of its behavior and mechanisms.

---

15 https://www.webmd.com/vitamins-and-supplements/quercetin-uses-and-risks

- Interactome and interactomics—the body of reactive species and the study of their interactions and downstream effects.
- Lipidome and lipidomics—the body of lipids in a cell, tissue, or organism and the study of their pathways and networks.
- Metabolome and metabolomics—the body of metabolites in a cell, tissue, or organism, and the study of their behavior.
- Metallome and Metallomics—the body of metal ions in tissue or cells.
- Microbiome and microbiomics—the body of microbes on the epithelium or in a part of the body, such as the intestines.
- Proteome and proteomics—the body of proteins in a cell, tissue, or organism.
- Secretome and secretomics—the body of secreted proteins and their behavior and mechanisms.
- Transcriptome and transcriptomics—the body of RNA transcripts and the study of their role in genetic expression and regulation.
- Multi-omics—the application of a cross-section of the above -omics fields in the study of a discipline or topic (e.g., redox biology)
- And many, many, more.

This explosion of -omics fields and associated tools and techniques not only dramatically increased our ability to understand how the body and disease work but also sped it up. For example, the record turnaround of viable COVID-19 vaccines in 2020 was largely attributable to -omics technologies like PCR (polymerase chain reaction) that have dramatically increased our ability to study and understand RNA and microRNA behaviors. The impact of -omics on epistemology is that this explosion of knowledge about how the body works biochemically is disproportionately occurring at the low-end of the evidence hierarchy.

From a medical perspective, if you prove that a medicine works in a mouse, you haven't proven that it works in a human, and thus it's considered low-quality evidence. But if you demonstrate that a medicine upregulates the NRF2 pathway in a mouse and by extension activates hundreds of genes related to cellular defense, the likelihood that it will behave similarly in humans is very high because biochemically, humans, mice, and even plants share an astonishing amount of chemistry, processes, and even systems. Suddenly, those "low-end" studies become much more important because they help you understand complex systems and how they behave and interact. At some point, these low-end studies begin to critique your earlier high-end randomized controlled clinical trials. Knowledge of how complex systems actually work leads to better treatment paradigms, and ultimately new and better treatment protocols.

There are many examples where studies showing how a system works trump and ultimately overturn the prevailing understanding. In the 1990s, the gastrointestinal tract was viewed as dumb plumbing even by gastroenterologists. In the 2000s, it became clear that the microbiome played important signaling functions and regulatory roles in every organ system. Similarly, to this day, there are GI doctors who doubt that intestinal permeability (aka leaky gut syndrome) is real. But in the early 2000s, researchers studying celiac disease were inducing it and curing it in mice and discovered the protein zonulin regulated intestinal tight junctions that determined what could pass through the intestinal barrier. When the intestinal barrier is hyperpermeable (leaky), endotoxin from the cell walls of dead gram-negative gut bacteria pass through the gut barrier and/or gut-vascular barrier and into the bloodstream where it powerfully activates the immune system, causing systemic inflammation. That's a problem, and it's called endotoxemia, a form of low-grade sepsis.

There will be many other examples throughout this book. Still, the key point is that you ultimately need both 1) observational, animal, and cell studies that demonstrate how bodily systems and disease processes work and 2) randomized clinical trials that prove the efficacy of specific therapies in human populations.

Quercetin has Multi-target Effects

In the 1990s, the drug development paradigm was "one gene, one target, one drug."[16] However, two decades later, researchers acknowledged that in the face of complex multi-factor diseases like Alzheimer's, the approach had failed, and a multitarget approach was needed. Interestingly, they looked to plant compounds like berberine and quercetin as models. Both quercetin and berberine activate both AMPK and NRF2 pathways. AMPK plays a primary role in regulating metabolism, and NRF2 upregulates cellular defenses and antioxidant status. Together they affect about 800 downstream genes, and though it's a generalization, I think it's fair to characterize AMPK and NRF2 as stress resilience pathways. Thus these epigenetic modifications are overwhelmingly positive and designed to help the organism restore and maintain homeostasis in the face of a wide range of stressors.

Quercetin is a Eustressor

While you may read about quercetin's free radical scavenging abilities, its primary mode of action is actually as a mild oxidant that, as stated previously, stimulates AMPK and NRF2, promoting an increase in cellular defenses. This is a phenomenon called eustress or hormesis, where a low-level stressor invokes a useful adaptive response, in this case, resistance to current stress and increased resilience to future stress. The key takeaway here is that you cannot understand the benefits of quercetin (or any other polyphenol) apart from redox biology's concept of eustress and the associated adaptive stress response.

---

16 Dias, Kris Simone Tranches, and Claudio Viegas Jr. "Multi-Target Directed Drugs: A Modern Approach for Design of New Drugs for the treatment of Alzheimer's Disease." *Current neuropharmacology* vol. 12,3 (2014): 239-55. doi:10.2174/1570159X1203140511153200

Summing up the Epistemological Problem

Quercetin nicely illustrates our current reality: we now have the tools and techniques to take things that we know work (e.g., plant-based diets) and identify useful components (e.g., quercetin), and then analyze in great detail how and why they work. In the process, we gain important insights into how complex bodily systems work in many scenarios and conditions. The epistemological problem is that these studies are largely animal, cell, and observational studies. In a rigidly orthodox western medical worldview, you are open to criticism that you have weak or no evidence. Thus, in an ironic twist, evidence-based medicine devalues or even rejects a large body of important evidence that would help improve health outcomes and move us closer to a personalized or precision medicine paradigm. That observation applies not only to quercetin but more broadly to research into oxidative stress and redox imbalance as root causes of disease.

I would submit that this rigidly orthodox view of evidence is simultaneously EBM's great strength, and in the 21st century, an even greater flaw. In a world where you really couldn't fully understand how the body or a therapy worked at a biochemical level, the EBM hierarchy of evidence protected us from therapies that were ineffective or dangerous and from quackery. Indeed, whether or not it was designed to do this, the EBM hierarchy of evidence has been used to exclude and denigrate "alternative medicine" modalities as non-scientific and ineffective. Scientific research shows us how the body—its systems and processes—work and how they break down under the stresses of aging and daily life. In the new reality, we can gather prodigious amounts of diverse biochemical data. Continuously monitoring key biomarkers is increasingly feasible and cost-effective. Thus, the therapeutic goals could be to optimize your nutritional status, redox status, immune status, and epigenetic status rather than managing a specific disease or symptom.

These tools can be used to evaluate current therapies and assumptions and even apply to alternative medicine paradigms such as Chinese Traditional Medicine, Ayurveda, chiropractic, and other ethnomedicine traditions. The EBM evidence hierarchy, designed to be slow, safe, and conservative, now threatens to inhibit our ability to rapidly adopt new ideas and paradigms and treatment modalities such as personalized or precision medicine, personalized nutrition, and personalized therapies. It impedes our ability to shed or modify outdated protocols and puts core disciplines like nutrition outside of the medical paradigm. And it impedes our ability to learn from the medical wisdom of other cultures. I would argue that this is not inherent in the evidence hierarchy but is rather an abuse of the evidence hierarchy in defense of the EBM status quo.

Precision Medicine and EBM Evidence Hierarchy

Ever since the sequencing of the human genome, the prospect of personalized or precision medicine has tantalized the world of western medicine. Through a combination of genetic information about an individual patient and information about their current health status, nutritional status, immune status, redox status, epigenetic status, various other relevant biomarkers, and even the patient's beliefs and preferences, doctors could tailor specific treatments to a patient not only to treat disease symptoms after their onset but to prevent disease from occurring in the first place. That this is a different paradigm from traditional evidence-based medicine is acknowledged even by WebMD, a site that positions itself as authoritative for EBM health information. In a WebMD article entitled "Traditional vs. Precision Medicine: How They Differ," the author contrasts the two approaches:

"Traditional medicine and precision medicine are two approaches doctors use to treat disease. They work in different ways.

Traditional medicine follows a one-size-fits-all approach. Drugs and other therapies are designed to treat large groups of people with the same disease — like diabetes or cancer.

They may factor in your sex, age, or weight, but overall, doctors base your treatment on what's most likely to work for everyone with a similar illness.

But not everyone responds to a treatment in the same way. Some drugs work very well for certain people. Others don't help at all or cause harmful side effects. Finding the exact drug that works for you can involve a lot of trial and error.

Precision medicine takes things a step further. Doctors use information about you—your genes, lifestyle, and environment—along with the characteristics of your disease to select treatments that are most likely to work for you. Because it's so closely tied to who you are, precision medicine is sometimes called personalized medicine."[17]

Though the author presents the two approaches as co-existing side-by-side, there are potential conflicts that need to be reconciled. First, the corpus of EBM treatment protocols is almost entirely based on an evidence hierarchy and methodologies designed to ensure that a protocol works for a population (average treatment effect), not an individual (individual treatment effect)—as the author says, one-size-fits-all. Numerous writers have pointed out that this can be addressed through a more rigorous analysis of sub-populations and what are known as N-1 clinical trials (aka trials of 1). More serious is what I believe to be an abuse of the evidence hierarchy, where EBM fundamentalists treat research lower on the evidence hierarchy as "no evidence." I've encountered this numerous times on patient forums, where I'd be trying to figure out how a particular system worked based on the latest research and would be attacked by someone who claimed I "had no evidence." I was initially confused by this because I had LOTS of evidence. I finally realized that for these people, the position on the evidence hierarchy trumped understanding how the system actually worked, which is backwards.

---

17 Martin, Laura J. "Precision Medicine: How Is It Different From Traditional Medicine?" WebMD, WebMD, 9 June 2019, www.webmd.com/cancer/precision-vs-traditional-medicine.

I believe the solution to the above problem is for evidence-based medicine to be explicitly based on systems biology, multi-omics methodologies, and a commitment to understanding how systems and therapies work at a molecular level. This would set up a virtuous circle, where understanding how bodily systems, diseases, and therapies work helps critique and improve existing therapeutic protocols, shed those that are outmoded, and create new and better protocols. In return, increasingly high-quality evidence provides ever clearer and more detailed models for how the systems work and validates emerging therapies based on the latest understandings. If that happens, then I believe that traditional EBM and precision medicine can indeed co-exist and benefit each other as EBM essentially *becomes* precision medicine. The patient will be the winner.

In subsequent chapters, you will periodically find things that may look like a critique of western medicine. This is largely because I view redox imbalance and its treatment as, by definition, a manifestation of precision medicine/personalized medicine and redox biology and research into redox systems as a gateway to precision medicine. Redox biologists, geneticists, and others plying multi-omics techniques are showing us how the body works. My critiques are primarily to point out what I think are opportunities to apply those learnings to improve medicine and empower patients. We will revisit these ideas in future chapters, but first, we need to take a deeper dive into the world of redox imbalance, the disease we don't measure, diagnose, or treat.

Chapter 4

Redox Imbalance: The Disease We Don't Treat

"Natural forces within us are the true healers of disease."

—Hippocrates

The idea that there is a root cause of disease is sure to meet with some degree of skepticism. However, if you were to design such a root cause, you'd probably tie it to some foundational process, like respiration, that affects every cell in the body. And if you tied it to some universal electrochemical process like electron transfer that underlies every chemical process in the body, that would be truly ingenious. And if you positioned this mechanism at the nexus of the genetic machinery and the environmental stressors that necessitate adaptation, well, that would be incredibly elegant. I've just described the body's redox mechanisms and stress response systems, which protect you from the daily onslaught of stressors, make useful adaptations but can be damaged, overwhelmed, and dysregulated by chronic or extreme stress. The result is disease and associated symptoms.

Redox Imbalance versus Oxidative Stress

Given that the lion's share of the research into redox imbalance is on oxidative stress, why not just call it oxidative stress?

Good question. Up until recently, oxidative stress was the prevalent way scientists talked about redox imbalance. You may have even heard of things like the oxidative stress theory of aging, preceded by Harman's free radical theory of aging. As science has advanced, the old descriptors were found to be inadequate or inaccurate for two key reasons:
1. Researchers discovered that oxidative stress was actually beneficial at low levels, a phenomenon known as hormesis or eustress (meaning good stress).
2. They also discovered that reductive stress was real and affected metabolic regulation via depletion of NAD+, an oxidant.

These two discoveries made it clear that oxidative stress was not sufficiently accurate to describe the health impacts of redox homeostasis gone wrong. Oxidative stress and diminished antioxidant capacity are still real and important. Still, like it or not, redox imbalance is the best phrase to describe the totality of what's going on in disease states.

Redox Imbalance *Is* the Disease

With the help of a legion of scientists, I am making the case that imbalance in the body's redox defense and regulatory systems is a root cause of most disease, chronic and acute. The scientists are brilliant and the evidence compelling, but sometimes a good metaphor is more effective at making a new idea like 'redox imbalance is a disease' stick. So consider the saga of my humble freezer:

In my garage was a small freezer stocked with frozen veggies, meat, and other items that didn't fit in the kitchen fridge freezer. It was designed to keep those items at about 0° Fahrenheit, with a compressor to pump the coolant through the coils, heat coils on the back to exhaust the heat from the interior, a thermostat to regulate the temperature, insulation to keep the heat out and the cold in, and a rubber gasket on the door to seal in the cold air in when it was shut. One day I noticed water on the garage floor and assumed it was from the car, as we'd had some snow recently. Many trips to the garage later, I went to get something from the freezer and discovered that it was WARM! The door had been slightly ajar for about two days, all the food was thawed, the coils were defrosted, the compressor had burned up, and the freezer was kaput.

In the metaphor, my freezer developed a case of 'open door disease' where the open door was the source of the stress, which caused loss of thermal (redox) homeostasis. Sensors in the thermostat detected the problem and invoked an adaptive response—firing up the compressor to lower the temperature. However, the heat loss was too great for the compressor to overcome, so it constantly ran until it failed (sudden compressor death)—the freezer and its contents lost. To push the analogy further, in the western medical paradigm, we'd focus all our attention on the compressor (compressor disease!) and how to keep it from failing, while in a redox imbalance paradigm, we'd shut the door. It's also worth pointing out that in my example, had I shut the door when I first noticed the water, I would have prevented the entire cascade of warming freezer, failing compressor, thawing/spoiling food, and dead freezer. It's a cautionary tale that highlights the importance of treating root causes.

While your body is vastly more complicated than my freezer, the same basic principles apply.

As stated earlier, in epidemiological terms, redox imbalance is an insufficient but necessary cause in all disease. By extension, **redox imbalance *is* a disease**. With a compelling and growing body of evidence, the reality that redox imbalance is not *already* considered a disease in mainstream medical practice says volumes about the entrenched nature of the current disease paradigm and the disconnect between the body of therapeutic protocols and the rapidly evolving understanding of how the body works.

Allowing that disease status for redox imbalance is not going to happen without significant resistance, let us consider what things might look like if it were the case:

1. We would establish routine biomarkers and tests to measure redox imbalance.
2. We would identify root cause stressors and mitigate them.
3. We would establish routine tests to measure the common nutritional deficits associated with oxidative stress.
4. We would develop more effective testing methodologies for identifying hidden or chronic low-grade infection, a common source of oxidative stress and inflammation.
5. We would establish dietary guidelines that help maintain optimal redox status.
6. We would establish helpful self-care guidelines for sleep, exercise, and stress management to maintain redox balance.
7. We would identify useful protocols for over-the-counter optimization of the immune system and stopping early-stage infections.
8. We would develop more powerful medical therapies for reestablishing redox balance in extreme or advanced cases.
9. Existing disease treatment protocols would be reconsidered in light of their impact on redox status, nutritional status, immune status, gut microbiome homeostasis, metabolic status, and epigenetic impact. Outmoded, ineffective, or injurious protocols would be replaced by more effective ones.
10. Medicines that raise oxidative or reductive stress levels would be particularly suspect.
11. Agricultural policy would shift towards incentivizing cost-effective production of fruits, vegetables, and other nutrient-dense foods.
12. Consumer demand would shift away from highly-processed grains, sugar, omega-6 oils, and preservative-laden foods toward minimally processed and whole foods.
13. We would establish maintenance, therapeutic, and upper-limit, not-to-exceed levels for key nutritional supplements since high levels often have diminishing returns and even negative consequences.

14. We would continue to strengthen clean air and water standards to reduce exposure to particulates, toxins, and xenobiotics.

If this seems like pie-in-the-sky, fantasy thinking, consider that the seeds of this revolution are already sown. Soft drink sales have experienced ten years of declining sales.[18] In 2015, General Mills shut down two plants to adjust to consumer behavior, shifting away from packaged breakfast foods.[19] Many health consumers have already adopted alternative treatment strategies outside standard paradigms—from supplements to acupuncture to chiropractic. While some concerns accompany this trend (i.e., quackery and efficacy), it puts consumer pressure on the medical establishment to raise its game and get better. Most importantly, the scientific research supporting the shift is publicly available in free abstracts or, in many cases, full-text form.

Earlier I stated that redox imbalance is both the insufficient but necessary cause in all disease and redox imbalance is the disease, hence the book's title! While these two statements may appear to have the potential for conflict, I see both synergy and profound implications. Consider:
- If redox imbalance is a disease, you measure, diagnose, and treat it. In doing so, you are, in effect, treating all disease, current, and future.
- If redox imbalance is a disease caused by stress, you care a lot about the potential sources of stress and how to eliminate, mitigate, or manage them. If you can accomplish this, you will prevent or reduce the incidence of all disease.
- If loss of stress resilience is a clinical feature of redox imbalance (and it is), then it's a high therapeutic value to bolster or restore that resilience. If you can accomplish this, you will prevent or alleviate many symptoms and comorbid diseases.

---

18 Soft Drinks Hit 10th Year of Decline, *Wall Street Journal,* March 26, 2015
19 General Mills to Close 2 Plants, Cut More Than 600 Jobs, *Wall Street Journal,* July 16, 2015

- If redox imbalance causes downstream damage and systemic dysregulation that manifests itself as symptoms and comorbid diseases then that progression can be described, and interventions designed to prevent it.

To fully engage these and other implications, we will need to master some foundational concepts behind redox imbalance.

Redox Imbalance: Foundational Concepts

Accepting that redox imbalance is a root cause of disease is a fundamentally different paradigm from traditional western medicine. And as pointed out in the previous chapter, it is more aligned with precision medicine/personalized medicine because the very notion of eustress and distress is contextual. It's going to be different for every patient and different for the same patient at different periods in their life. Running a 5K, which would generally be thought of as a eustressor, is a morning jog for one person and likely to cause permanent damage to a second person. That second person, with six months of training, might be out running marathons.

Every paradigm and discipline has its foundational concepts and associated jargon—no surprise there. If you want to benefit from the new paradigm, it's useful and often necessary to learn them. The remainder of this chapter is devoted to exploring what I consider to be foundational for understanding redox imbalance as a disease and as a biochemical phenomenon affecting not just humans but all life on this planet. While redox imbalance is a complex and evolving topic, understanding it necessarily begins with oxidative stress.

Concept: Oxidative Stress

In 1985, Helmut Sies published a book entitled "Oxidative Stress," a collection of 18 scientific articles that framed oxidative stress as "a disturbance in the pro-oxidant/antioxidant systems in favour of the former." Initial research focused on oxidative damage by free radicals (e.g., superoxide, hydrogen peroxide, and the hydroxyl radical) to proteins, lipids, carbohydrates, and DNA. However, in the last two decades, the research emphasis has shifted to the signaling role of a much broader range of reactive species catalyzed by those initial free radicals. Along with that, research has come to a far more nuanced view of oxidative stress—that the body is designed to function with and benefit from low levels of oxidative stress, termed **eustress** (meaning "good stress"). In tandem, the original concept of oxidative stress as damage emanating from chronic or excessive production of reactive species evolved to include dysregulated/pathological signaling and reframed as **distress** (meaning "bad stress"). Whether oxidative stress is eustress or distress is highly contextual. A vigorous workout could kill or injure one person and benefit another. That principle extends to a broader range of therapies, including existing medical protocols not currently understood as redox therapies.

Concept: Redox Pools

All living things have developed complex systems for maintaining redox homeostasis. For humans, we're going to focus on what are known as redox pools. Each pool is composed of a redox couple: two chemical compounds, one reduced, one oxidized. Each pool has systems of enzymes and raw materials known as precursors and co-factors that maintain the pool's size and oxidative state. The state of the pool is either oxidized or reduced. The human redox pools include

- **The glutathione pool**, the primary intracellular redox pool, is composed of the GSH/GSSG redox couple. GSH is reduced glutathione, and GSSG is the oxidized form. The glutathione pool needs to be maintained in a reduced state for healthy cellular function and antioxidant defense.

A depleted or oxidized glutathione pool is associated with reduced antioxidant capacity and reduced stress resilience and is commonly found in aging and disease states.

- **The NADP pool** plays a key role in maintaining the glutathione and thioredoxin pools and is composed of the NADP+/NADPH redox couple. NADP+ is the oxidized form, while NADPH is reduced. The NADP pool needs to be maintained in a reduced state. An oxidized or depleted NADP pool is associated with elevated ROS production and oxidative stress and loss of antioxidant capacity and stress resilience.
- **The NAD pool** is associated with electron transport, energy production, DNA repair, and regulation of the cell's mitochondria and is comprised of the NAD+/NADH redox couple. NAD+ is the oxidized form, and NADH is reduced. The NAD pool needs to be maintained in an oxidized state. A depleted or reduced NAD pool will result in diminished energy production and impaired DNA repair and is commonly found in aging and disease states.
- **The cysteine pool** is increasingly appreciated as an important set of redox switches found in the cytosol and sensitive to extracellular oxidative stress. The cysteine redox couple is composed of cysteine and cystine, often abbreviated as Cys/CySS, with cysteine being the reduced thiol form and cystine being oxidized disulfide form.

While there are other redox pools (e.g., thioredoxin), these four stand out as key to our understanding of redox health. Dysregulation of the NAD pool is key to understanding metabolic dysregulation, disordered energy production, and downstream diseases like heart disease and diabetes. Dysregulation of the NADP pool can dramatically increase ROS production and decrease levels of reduced glutathione (GSH). Dysregulation of the glutathione pool can reduce stress resilience as well as lower immune function and detoxification capacity. Dysregulation of the extracellular cysteine pool impacts intracellular redox status, and dysregulation of intracellular cysteine impacts protein function and signaling.

Because of their central role in energy production and stress resilience, these redox pools are also promising therapeutic targets in treating a wide variety of diseases. More on that later.

Concept: The Redox Code

In their 2015 article, "The Redox Code,"[20] authors Sies and Jones describe a redox code analogous and complementary to the genetic code, epigenetic code[21], and histone code[22] for understanding "the molecular logic of life." Using an analogy to computer hardware/software, the genetic code and histone code function as hardware for storing and transmitting biological information, while the epigenetic code and redox code function as software, defining the operation of the underlying genetic and histone codes in the "organizational structure, differentiation, and adaptation of an organism to the environment." In this framework, redox systems, mechanisms and status are essential to our understanding of how organisms—their cells and systems, their health, disease, and life cycles—work. The redox code has four principles that underlie the organization of biological systems:

1. **Nicotinamide, with its reversible electron-accepting and donating properties, is integral to metabolism**. This is manifested in NAD and NADP systems, operating at near equilibrium, which play organizing and regulatory roles in energy production, anabolism (metabolism that synthesizes complex molecules from simpler ones), and catabolism (metabolism that breaks down complex molecules into simpler ones, releasing energy).

---

20 Jones, Dean P, and Helmut Sies. "The Redox Code." *Antioxidants & redox signaling* vol. 23,9 (2015): 734-46. doi:10.1089/ars.2015.6247

21 Bhan, A., Deb, P. and Mandal, S.S. "Epigenetic Code. In Gene Regulation, Epigenetics and Hormone Signaling," S.S. Mandal (Ed.) (2017): doi:10.1002/9783527697274.ch2

22 Shahid Z, Simpson B, Miao KH, et al. "Genetics, Histone Code." [Updated 2020 Sep 2]. In: StatPearls [Internet]. Treasure Island (FL): StatPearls Publishing; 2020 Jan.

2. **The Redox Proteome links metabolism with chemical structure via redox switches**, typically sulfur thiols, which are easily switched between thiol and disulfide states. These switches determine macromolecules' activity, movement, and function (e.g., proteins, DNA). In perhaps overly simplistic terms, you can think of this principle and the related system as maintaining and regulating the redox proteome via cysteine and methionine redox switches that are controlled by H_2O_2 (oxidation) and glutathione and thioredoxin (reduction), all with implications for redox sensing and signaling, protein production and function, and cellular differentiation, expression and life cycle.

3. **Activation/deactivation cycles of H_2O_2 facilitate redox sensing and signaling systems that regulate cellular expression, differentiation, and life cycles**, facilitating the development of multicellular organisms. In a follow-on article, Sies describes the central role of H_2O_2 as a redox signaling molecule, whose concentration in serum ultimately governs whether oxidative stress/oxidative signaling functions as eustress or pathological distress.[23]

4. **The body's redox networks form an adaptive system that allows an organism and its cells to adapt to environmental stressors.** These networks operate at sub-cellular, cellular, tissue, and system levels. This principle implies that the redox system's dysregulation and/or failure contributes to disease and ultimately death.

As you can see from the above four points, "The Redox Code" is a dense piece of work, so don't be discouraged if you don't understand it. Its significance is that it corrals the growing body of redox research into a concise yet powerful, conceptual biochemical framework. That framework places redox systems and processes at the foundation of virtually

---

23 Sies, Helmut. "Hydrogen peroxide as a central redox signaling molecule in physiological oxidative stress: Oxidative eustress." Redox biology vol. 11 (2017): 613-619. doi:10.1016/j.redox.2016.12.035

every process related to the function, regulation, and life cycle of cells, systems, and organisms with profound health and disease implications.

Concept: The Cellular Stress Response

At the top of the Redox Disease Model are a list of stress inputs. There is a foundational principle underlying this list: namely, that a body and its cells, under stress, produce increased quantities of reactive oxygen and nitrogen species (ROS/RNS). At the base of this principle is the cellular stress response, which has been described in detail in multiple scientific papers.

In a 2018 article from *Nature Reviews* entitled "Linking cellular stress responses to systemic homeostasis,"[24] authors Galluzzi, Yamazaki, and Kroemer describe the cellular response to stress stimuli as consisting of:

- **The heat shock response:** Increased production of heat shock proteins is a cytoprotective response.
- **The unfolded protein response:** This mechanism acts to restore protein folding capacity in the endoplasmic reticulum.
- **The DNA damage response:** This mechanism attempts to repair damaged DNA and inhibit cellular replication of damaged or mutated DNA (i.e., cell cycle arrest).
- **Mitochondrial stress signaling:** Increased mitochondrial ROS production can lead to inflammasome activation and local inflammation, as well as a mitochondrial version of the unfolded protein response.
- **Autophagy:** Literally "self-eating," autophagy is a cellular recycling process that can operate at a subcellular level to clear irreversibly damaged cellular components and re-

---

[24] Galluzzi, Lorenzo et al. "Linking cellular stress responses to systemic homeostasis." Nature reviews. Molecular cell biology vol. 19,11 (2018): 731-745. doi:10.1038/s41580-018-0068-0

use the raw materials. Autophagy is typically induced by nutritional deficits, energy depletion, and oxidative stress. Successful autophagy can prevent regulated cell death, whereas dysregulated autophagy can induce cell death.

These adaptive stress responses are designed to restore homeostasis to stressed cells. If unsuccessful, cells are either deactivated (senescence) or destroyed via regulated cell death. The cellular stress response also includes extracellular danger signaling that evokes a systemic adaptive response designed to restore homeostasis at a system and organism level. Though useful, these responses can be maladaptive, leading to disease and death. Other research has shown that NRF2 activation, which you can think of as the oxidative stress response, plays a key role in upregulating heat shock protein production, enhancing DNA damage response signaling, and modulating the unfolded protein response. Similarly, the AMPK pathway is invoked in response to energy-related stress. These early adaptive responses then play a key role in the activation and regulation of the immune response—all supporting the core principle that redox processes are integral to all facets of the cellular stress response.

Cellular Stress Response: Key Takeaway

In the "cellular stress response," the body and its cells under stress produce increased quantities of reactive oxygen and nitrogen species. The resulting oxidative stress (OS) and downstream signaling is the foundational cellular warning signal that something is wrong. Thus, OS is well-positioned to be the foundational signaling initiator of the protective/adaptive response and the broader effort to maintain or restore homeostasis at a cellular, system, and organism level.

Concept: Genome/Exposome

If genetics set us up for vigorous debates about what could be attributed to heredity and what is due to environment, the field of epigenetics gave us a scientific framework for thinking about the impact of environmental exposure on genetic expression.

While the concept of the genome, a collection of genetic information that is fixed, is well-known, the exposome is a new concept for many of us. The idea of the exposome is that each of us has a genome that is fixed and analogous to computer hardware, but we also each have experiences that shape the expression of those genes. Those collective experiences are known as the exposome and are analogous to software in that they shape how the hardware behaves. A key concept in the exposome is that early life experiences have both great significance and potentially long-term impact on health and well-being.

Examples of early-life exposures with long-term impact include shaken-baby syndrome or fetal alcohol syndrome, or on the positive side, breastfeeding.

Redox biology has embraced the idea of the genome-exposome and proposed that redox systems serve as the interface between the genome and the exposome. Research into the cellular stress response, and signaling pathways such as NRF2, AMPK, FOXO, PGC1a and HO-1, support this concept.

Concept: Cumulative Stress Load

This book promotes the understanding that stress and oxidative stress are derived from a much broader range of sources than the traditional understanding of psychological stress. If you search for "cumulative stress load" on PubMed, you'll find many articles on allostasis and allostatic load. These are terms coined by neuropsychoendocrinologists McEwen, Eyer, Stellar, and others in the late 1980s and early 1990s as a corrective to perceived weaknesses in the homeostatic model of physiology, which many have viewed as rigid and mechanistic. In a 2003 article, John Wingfield describes allostasis and allostatic load in the following manner:

> "The concept of allostasis, maintaining stability through change, is a fundamental process through which organisms actively adjust to both predictable and unpredictable events... Allostatic load refers to the cumulative cost to the body of allostasis, with allostatic overload... being a state in which serious pathophysiology can occur."

Allostasis has become the most prominent of many alternate models to homeostasis. (For a deeper dive into allostasis and allostatic load, the 2014 article "Clarifying the Roles of Homeostasis and Allostasis in Physiological Regulation" gives a good overview.)

For our purposes, allostasis/allostatic load and cumulative stress load are virtually indistinguishable. They are a sign of convergence between redox biology and neuropsychoendocrinology, which began incorporating oxidative stress biomarkers into its scientific articles late in the first decade of the 2000s. While not widely known outside of the research world, these ideas and the Allostatic Load Index (ALI) have been around long enough that a 2020 article was able to quantify an increase in allostatic load between 2005 and 2018 for a racially diverse cohort of 26,818 participants. Not surprisingly, black and Latinx participants experienced a greater rise in allostatic load than US and foreign-born whites, with foreign-born blacks and foreign-born Latinx women experiencing the greatest erosion in health. The study concludes that

> "Chronic exposure to stressors leads to an erosion of health that is particularly severe among foreign-born Blacks and Latinx. Policies should seek to reduce exposure to structural and environmental risks and to ensure equitable

opportunities to achieve optimal health among racial/ethnic minorities and immigrants."[25]

The significance of such a study (and the Allostatic Load Index more broadly) is that it supports the idea that allostatic load/stress burden can be measured and that increased stress burden is associated with erosion of health.

In a clinical application of a redox health paradigm, doctors would help patients understand and think about what their cumulative stress load might be. Early in the treatment process, a doctor and patient would have an in-depth conversation about the stress inputs in the patient's life. These stressors are simultaneously the drivers of dysregulation and disease, and often the piece the patient has the most control over (though not always), so it makes sense to start there. Are you getting regular exercise? Adequate sleep? Eating a nutrient-dense diet? Under psychological, relational, or financial stress? Taking prescription medications? Had a recent infection? A physical injury? Chronic pain? A past trauma? Any allergies or rashes? Headaches? Digestive complaints? Other physical symptoms? For the patient, regardless of race, ethnicity, educational attainment, and economic status, finding ways to eliminate, mitigate, or manage the stressors in their life is an important contribution to their future health and wholeness.

While this is an important and useful conversation, we must also acknowledge that not everyone under stress gets sick, which leads us to the next concept: stress resilience.

Concept: Stress Resilience

Why do some people get cancer, depression, or other illnesses, and others don't? Why do older people get cancer and other illnesses at higher rates than their younger counterparts? The concept of stress resilience explains this. The tantalizing

---

25 Langellier, Brent A et al. "Allostatic Load Among U.S.- and Foreign-Born Whites, Blacks, and Latinx." American journal of preventive medicine, S0749-3797(20)30406-2. 26 Nov. 2020, doi:10.1016/j.amepre.2020.08.022

notion that we might be able to strengthen or restore that resilience is one of the more exciting ideas to emerge from the research behind this book.

In the theory of allostasis, coping with or adapting to a stressor incurs a "cost" to an organism, which can be understood in terms of redox-driven damage and dysregulation. This could help explain the general human resistance to even positive change. This coping/adaptation process requires healthy nutritional status, redox status, metabolic status, and immune status to work properly. The systems behind these functions should be understood as interdependent because they are. Consider:

- To make and recycle glutathione, your body needs nutrients: cysteine, glycine, glutamine, magnesium, vitamins B12 and D3, and lipoic acid.
- Glutathione has important immune functions—both regulatory functions and direct tasks like detoxification and inhibition of viral replication. Thus, low glutathione status impacts immune function.
- To make energy efficiently, your metabolism needs a healthy NAD+/NADH pool, and that requires nutrients (e.g., nicotinamide and taurine). Overconsumption of processed carbs, sugar, and fructose depletes NAD+, as does DNA damage from the overproduction of ROS by stressors or an overly active immune system.
- An inefficient metabolism overproduces ROS and underproduces the energy needed for cells and systems to function properly.

This list is in no way comprehensive but illustrates how these interrelated systems can support health but also spiral downward into damage, dysregulation, and disease.

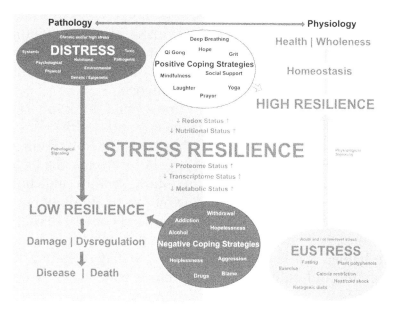

Stress resilience: a model

In the above model, distress, or negative stress, leads to low-stress resilience, damage, dysregulation, disease, and death. In contrast, eustress, or good stress, leads to enhanced stress resilience, homeostasis, health, and wholeness. Each person also has an individual collection of coping strategies that are either positive or negative and contribute to or subvert stress resilience. Finally, the text in the center shows stress resilience components that are either healthy or unhealthy, represented by the up or down arrows. Redox status refers to the balance between oxidation and reduction, while nutritional status addresses the availability of nutritional raw materials necessary for proper cellular and system function. Proteome status refers to the production of the proper proteins for each cell type, transcriptome status to the set of RNA messengers for appropriate gene expression, and metabolic status to the overall health of energy production and cellular mitochondria.

When we see stress resilience breaking down, it is often explainable by elevated cumulative stress load and inadequate low-level eustressors such as exercise, dietary plant polyphenols, and calorie restriction, along with sleep deficits and the loss of important antioxidant minerals, vitamins, and amino acids. Together, they reduce antioxidant capacity, redox buffering, lowered immune function, dysregulated metabolism, and lowered stress resilience.

Read that last paragraph a few times, and I think you'll agree that as you reflect on your own illnesses and health crises, you can often identify the stressors that contributed to them. One of the next tasks for medicine is to craft scientifically testable strategies and protocols that maintain, restore, and bolster your stress resilience, thereby avoiding or diminishing any illness's severity and/or duration. I am not content to wait and have already begun creating my own protocols that I believe have helped me keep chronic illness at bay despite a high-stress job and suboptimal compliance with my own health principles.

Concept: Threshold of Pathology

The threshold of pathology is a concept that helps explain symptoms that come and go. We've all likely experienced this in ourselves or others—a weather-change headache, an aging relative's cognitive decline in the evening (sundowning), a rash that comes and goes, sinus pain that's worse on high allergen days, depression that's worse at night, etc. I find it useful to think about this phenomenon: Both stress burden and stress resilience have a cyclical quality. They rise and fall daily, weekly, or seasonally, or based on events and stimuli. If the stress burden is too high and stress resilience too low, the lines cross at the threshold of pathology. At that point, you become symptomatic, as shown in the figure below. Figure A shows a cyclical symptomatic state, and Figure B shows a state of health.

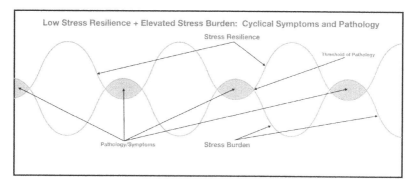

Figure A. Lowered stress resilience and cyclical symptoms and pathology

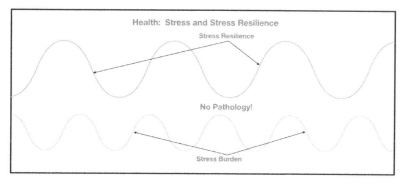

Figure B. Normal stress resilience and manageable stress burden

Concept: Disease Loops and Pro-Oxidant States

An emerging concept in understanding disease progression, drawn from systems theory, is the notion of feedforward loops. In a feedforward loop, a signal is sent in response to a stimulus, and no feedback response is required for the next signal to be sent. This is a very efficient signaling mechanism, but it can result in the self-sustaining, self-amplifying loops involved in inflammation, oxidative stress, and disease progression. There are also positive and negative feedback loops involved in regulating bodily processes that can become dysregulated, contributing to pro-oxidant states characterized by inflammation, pain, and other disease symptoms.

As we explore how oxidative stress/redox imbalance becomes disease, we are looking for these disease loops as mechanisms that both explain the initiation and progression of disease and give us potential targets for treating and resolving disease and associated symptoms. The science of identifying and understanding these disease loops is in its infancy, but also critically important to understanding how specific diseases work and how to treat them. Prediction: the most effective treatments will target the disease loops closest to their root cause.

Probable disease loops include

Oxidative Stress ➡ Magnesium Depletion 🔁

The idea of stress and magnesium forming a "vicious circle" dates back to the early 1990s.[26] Magnesium expulsion from the cell has been observed in restrained rat studies and is associated with stress hormones (e.g., catecholamines and cortisol). Low magnesium status prevents optimal glutathione status, which leads to increased oxidative stress (repeat). Diets rich in leafy greens, beans, nuts, and seeds help disrupt this loop, but magnesium supplementation may be necessary under high stress and when taking medications that deplete magnesium or block its absorption (e.g., fluoroquinolone antibiotics, proton pump inhibitors).

---

26 Pickering, Gisèle et al. "Magnesium Status and Stress: The Vicious Circle Concept Revisited." *Nutrients* vol. 12,12 3672. 28 Nov. 2020, doi:10.3390/nu12123672

Oxidative Stress ➡ NF-κB ➡ TNF-alpha 🔄

TNF-alpha is a major regulator of the inflammatory immune response, which results in increased ROS production. ROS activates the NF-κB pathway resulting in increased production of TNF-alpha (repeat). Various polyphenols and immune-related nutrients (e.g., zinc) have reasonable evidence for disrupting this loop.

Oxidative Stress ➡ Upregulation of Galectin-3 ➡ Upregulation of NADPH oxidase (NOX) Enzymes 🔄

Galectin-3 is a protein implicated in tissue fibrosis, insulin resistance, inflammation, Alzheimer's, cancer, heart failure, and other pathologies. Oxidative stress from stressors such as hypoxia upregulates galectin-3, which upregulates NOX enzymes leading to increased ROS (repeat). Modified citrus pectin[27] and curcumin[28] have been shown to inhibit galectin-3.

Oxidative stress ➡ Thiamine Deficiency ➡ Impaired Glucose Metabolism ➡ Increased Oxidative Stress 🔄

Thiamine deficiency is implicated in both diabetes and various neurodegenerative diseases. There is reasonable evidence to suggest that it participates in a pro-oxidant disease loop. Alcoholism, a prominent stressor, causes thiamine deficiency. Thiamine deficiency disrupts glucose metabolism and energy production leading to increased ROS production (repeat). Benfotiamine supplementation, a bioavailable form of thiamine, is an effective therapy for addressing thiamine deficiency. Benfotiamine supplementation has been shown

---

[27] Yin, Qingqing et al. "Pharmacological Inhibition of Galectin-3 Ameliorates Diabetes-Associated Cognitive Impairment, Oxidative Stress and Neuroinflammation in vivo and in vitro." *Journal of inflammation research* vol. 13 533-542. 15 Sep. 2020, doi:10.2147/JIR.S273858

[28] Dumi, Jerka et al. "Curcumin – A Potent Inhibitor of Galectin-3 Expression." (2005).

to be effective in preventing tissue damage in diabetes and improving cognitive impairment in old age.

There are far more of these disease loops than currently recognized. We can predict that we will find them where oxidative stress-driven nutritional deficiencies occur and in chronic activation of the HPA axis, sympathetic nervous system, renin-angiotensin-aldosterone system, immune system, and other pro-oxidant dysregulations such as mitochondrial dysfunction, gut dysbiosis, gut, and vascular permeability, and obesity.

Concept: Individual Stress Effect

A corollary of the cumulative stress load concept is what I refer to as the Individual Stress Effect. With cumulative stress load, you can visualize all your stressors piled up on an old-fashioned scales balanced against your antioxidant capacity/stress resilience/redox buffering capacity. It's a useful concept for understanding why too much stress would ultimately outstrip your ability to resolve or manage it and descend into disease. However, it falls short in helping us understand the impact of an individual stressor, which is where the individual stress effect concept comes in.

Every year when we turn our clocks forward in the spring, I can count on there being an article enumerating the health impacts of daylight saving time (DST), like this one from the New York Times: "Daylight Saving Time Takes a Toll on Health."[29] Turning our clocks forward is undoubtedly a stressor and one that results in some tangible health events, including heart attacks, hospitalizations, and even death, for a very small number of people every time we do it. If we use this one example to illustrate the idea of an individual stress effect, we might look at:

1. Magnitude. DST change is not a large stressor because most of us survive it every year.

---

29 https://www.nytimes.com/roomfordebate/2014/03/06/daylight-saving-time-at-what-cost/daylight-saving-time-takes-a-toll-on-health

2. Duration. Its impact can be measured in days. For example, accidental deaths are elevated for about a week after the spring clock change. So, not a long-term stressor, but not over in seconds either, like sneaking up behind someone and yelling, Boo!
3. Classification. An individual stress effect will vary from positive/eustress, to imperceptible, to negligible to noticeable, to annoying, to disabling, or even fatal. Spring clock change will affect sleep and circadian rhythms, and these typically fall into the category of distress. However, we can't rule out the idea of adaptive changes that make us more resilient to future DST changes.
4. Sufficiency. For a very small number of people, spring clock change is sufficient to trigger an adverse health event. Metaphorically, we'd say it's the straw that broke the camel's back—a very small thing that triggered a potentially catastrophic health event, typically a disease loop/pro-inflammatory cascade.
5. Context. The fact that the impacted number is very small says that an adverse individual stress effect or even a positive/eustress effect is contingent on the person and their context. Someone with a crushing cumulative stress load and loss of stress resilience is the metaphorical ticking time bomb. A small stressor is sufficient to 'push them over the edge,' 'cause them to snap,' 'send them into a downward spiral.' Linguistically, we could go on for pages enumerating the ways we talk about this phenomenon. But it mirrors the idea of a disease loop or pro-inflammatory cascade, where health status declines and sometimes declines very rapidly.

While there's more to say about this phenomenon, I'll leave you with the observation that eustressors can coexist with a heavy stress load and still provide adaptive benefits against current and future stress. We see this with exercise, saunas, plant-based diets, and other common eustressors. Conversely, something commonly assumed to be a eustressor, such as a treadmill workout, can also be a sufficient cause to trigger an adverse health effect (e.g., a heart attack).

In the end, the individual stress effect concept helps drive home that your goal should be to develop and maintain sufficient stress resilience such that no individual stressor becomes the sufficient cause for an adverse health event. That will entail both mitigating and managing our stress effectively through positive coping strategies and developing a robust collection of habits that promote resilience—topics we'll cover in more detail in upcoming chapters.

Summing Up

Thus far, we've introduced redox imbalance as both a new disease and the "insufficient but necessary cause" in every disease—in effect, a root cause of disease. We've followed the evolution of the science behind redox imbalance from Hans Selye's pioneering work on stress in the 1930s to free radical biology in the 1950s and the early emphasis on oxidative damage and antioxidants, to the introduction of oxidative stress in the 1980s and the current shift to redox signaling and a more nuanced view of oxidative stress that includes reductive stress and the notion of eustress and distress. Finally, in the current chapter, we've walked through the foundational concepts of redox imbalance: the cellular stress response, the genome and the exposome, cumulative stress load and stress resilience, the threshold of pathology, and disease loops.

The emerging picture is one where redox systems mediate a wide variety of stressors weighing on a person. They do so in ways that either maintain health and homeostasis through useful adaptations or degrade stress resilience and are ultimately overwhelmed, leading to damage, dysregulation of bodily systems, disease, and even death. While there is a great deal of complexity behind this scientific perspective, there is also a growing body of evidence indicating that we can bolster redox status and stress resilience with profound implications for slowing, reversing, and even curing diseases of all kinds. Before we move ahead with that exploration, we need to acknowledge that other important "component causes" are vying for our attention and give them due diligence.

Chapter 5

Redox Imbalance and the Case for Other Root Causes

Hippocrates postulated that an imbalance in the four humors—yellow bile, black bile, phlegm, and blood— was the root cause of disease. In the middle ages, "miasmas" or toxic vapors from cesspools, rotting carcasses, garbage, and other noxious sources, were thought to enter the body and cause disease. Germ theory superseded miasmas in the nineteenth century, and today public health researchers think in terms of "webs of causation" rather than any one single root cause.

Redox imbalance, in some ways, brings the notion of root cause mechanisms and a "web of causation" together. The idea is that the universal stress response, where cells under any stress produce reactive oxygen and nitrogen species, becomes the root cause, while the wildly diverse collection of stressors and the downstream pathologies become the "web of causation." I find this compelling because it explains phenomena that we've all experienced or wondered about, such as weather-change headaches and full-moon behavior at the elementary schools and nursing homes, as well as predicting behaviors for new phenomena, e.g., whether vaping would cause health problems (it should and it does).

But redox imbalance is not the only potential root cause issue vying for public attention or even the most prominent. While I am confident that redox imbalance belongs at the top of any root cause list, several other candidates deserve mention.

Root Cause Candidate 1: Genetics/Epigenetics and Anti-Aging Research

Ever since the sequencing of the human genome in April 2003, the idea that it would usher in a new era of personalized medicine has loomed as inevitable in the popular perception. The reality has proven much more complicated and elusive. It turns out we are a complex collection of genetic traits, often with overlapping, redundant, and even conflicting coding. Furthermore, the most relevant truth about genetics is that dynamic, epigenetic control of gene expression turns out to be the dominant theme in the medical application of genomic information. We adapt continuously to our environment. Genetic determinism is a relatively minor theme, and "bad" genes can go a lifetime without ever getting switched on.

A fruitful branch of genetic/epigenetic research is the field of anti-aging research. In his recent book *Lifespan*, biologist David Andrew Sinclair likens genetics to hardware, epigenetics to software, and aging to the scratched DVD that eventually becomes unreadable. While Sinclair rather casually brushes off the antioxidant theory of aging early in his book, I think it's fair to say that oxidative processes are certainly one of the main things that "scratch the epigenetic DVD." One of the main contributions of anti-aging research thus far is identifying useful compounds and strategies that generally reverse the loss of epigenetic information, with the tantalizing promise of making cells young again. Some of the most promising developments include

- Calorie restriction and intermittent fasting.
- Methionine-restricted diets (which provide another theoretical plank for the benefit of vegan diets).
- Drugs such as metformin and rapamycin.
- Supplements, including berberine, resveratrol, and pterostilbene.
- NAD+ repletion strategies including nicotinamide mononucleotide and nicotinamide riboside.
- Heat and cold stress.

- A heightened appreciation for cellular senescence in aging and certain disease pathologies and the role of senolytics (a new class of drugs or natural compounds that kill "death-resistant cells") as a potential strategy for slowing or reversing senescence.
- The discovery that many senolytic compounds protect normal cells while inducing senescence in tumor cells (e.g., fisetin, quercetin)[30]

The relationship between epigenetics and oxidative stress is that redox signaling is an important mechanism in epigenetic regulation of gene expression. Pathological genetic expression becomes just another mechanism for redox imbalance to cause disease. The epigenetic machinery also gives us therapeutic mechanisms—protective levers to pull, such as NRF2, AMPK, HO-1, PGC1a, and SIRT1, that can protect us from damage, dysregulation, and disease and reregulate damaged systems.

Genetics/Epigenetics and Anti-Aging Research: Key Takeaways

- Genetics and epigenetics play an undeniable role in determining how the body breaks down under stress/oxidative stress.
- Common epigenetic mechanisms are available as therapeutic tools for fighting disease. These include but are certainly not limited to KEAP1, NRF2, AMPK, and SIRT1. Genes like NRF2 and AMPK regulate potentially hundreds of other protective genes.
- We have evolved to benefit from the day-to-day microstressors, such as physical activity, fasting, commensal bacteria in the food we eat, and the low-level

---

[30] Malavolta, Marco et al. "Inducers of Senescence, Toxic Compounds, and Senolytics: The Multiple Faces of Nrf2-Activating Phytochemicals in Cancer Adjuvant Therapy." *Mediators of inflammation* vol. 2018 4159013. 12 Feb. 2018, doi:10.1155/2018/4159013

toxins in plants (e.g., polyphenols). Polyphenols and other phytonutrients are good examples of beneficial, low-level oxidative stressors.
- While the pharmaceutical industry has copied and modified plant chemistry to make prescription drugs, the reality is that our bodies are likely already designed to deal with the plant version and hence less likely to experience side effects from it. While there are exceptions to this observation, the relatively low level of side effects from plant polyphenols gives credence to this notion.
- I would predict increasing overlap and synergy between redox health and anti-aging research communities in the coming years. After all, increased lifespan without increased healthspan is pointless. All the anti-aging strategies in the world in the presence of chronic redox imbalance won't stop its corrosive, dysregulating effects.

Root Cause Candidate 2: The Microbiome

While I have yet to encounter an NPR news spot on redox imbalance, the microbiome seems to have captured popular attention in the health journalism world. This is perhaps because fecal transplants are both icky/attention-grabbing and have proven more effective for treating the notoriously stubborn hospital infection *C. difficile* than traditional antibiotic treatments. The microbiome is undeniably important, and understanding the role our bacterial partners play in the areas of signaling, immune function, inflammation, and disease goes hand-in-hand with understanding redox imbalance. Indeed, we should expect that anything with a shot at being a root cause issue will be integrally linked to oxidative stress.

For the microbiome, consider the following:

- "Good" bacteria (commensals) often produce hydrogen peroxide (H_2O_2), a prominent reactive oxygen species, which kills or suppresses "bad" (gram-negative) bacteria. This is why sauerkraut can ferment for weeks at room temperature and not make you sick. It contains its own *Lactobacillus plantarum*, which multiplies, producing H_2O_2 and killing off the competitors.
- Good bacteria help maintain the gut barrier, which keeps the bacterial toxin lipopolysaccharide (LPS) and other pathogenic and toxic stressors out of the bloodstream. If LPS gets into the bloodstream, it is a powerful oxidative stressor and activator of the immune system that will cause systemic inflammation and an additional layer of oxidative stress.
- A dysregulated oral microbiome can be a source of endotoxemia and whole-body inflammation (e.g., periodontitis), resulting in atherosclerosis, joint pain, and other inflammatory symptoms.
- Staph infection on the skin (a microbiome dysregulation by definition) produces a toxin called α-hemolysin or α-toxin that activates the immune system (via oxidative

stress), causing it to produce IL-17a. This inflammatory compound can cause a skin rash.
- The microbiome can play a role in causing obesity, and that metabolically active visceral fat, in turn, causes ongoing oxidative stress and inflammation through increased cytokine production.
- Oxidative stress-inducing dietary choices (high omega-6/trans fat diet, high fructose diet, sucralose, etc.) also encourage the growth of the wrong microbial tenants, changing the microbiome for the worse.
- Plant polyphenols and other NRF2 stimulators tend to change the gut microbiome for the better.
- Vitamin D3 status tracks with microbiome health.
- Mycotoxins produced by fungi such as *Candida albicans* and black mold are oxidative stressors and can cause cancer and contribute to other chronic ailments.
- There's a bidirectional relationship between the microbiome and oxidative stress (a feedforward loop), in which oxidative stress can dysregulate the microbiome. A dysregulated microbiome can, in turn, cause oxidative stress by degrading the gut barrier, dysregulating the immune system, causing increased vascular permeability, etc.

The Microbiome: Key Takeaways

A healthy, balanced microbiome will help protect you from oxidative stress-driven inflammation and chronic disease by:
- Maintaining the gut barrier, thus keeping bacteria and their toxic byproducts in the gut and out of the bloodstream.
- Checking the growth of pathogenic bacteria/viruses/fungi and their toxic byproducts.
- Digesting and metabolizing nutrients into useful, absorbable forms.
- Providing healthy signaling and regulation of other organ systems.
- Promoting a healthy, well-regulated immune system.
- Producing hormones and neurotransmitters (e.g., serotonin, dopamine) that support good mental health.

An unhealthy microbiome will exacerbate oxidative stress-driven inflammation and chronic disease by:

- Promoting intestinal permeability, which leads to the leakage of endotoxin into the bloodstream with resulting systemic inflammation.
- Allowing gut bacteria and bacterial byproducts into the bloodstream via increased vascular permeability can cause chronic low-grade infections at remote sites, such as the bladder and urinary tract.
- Under-producing certain key nutrients like B vitamins.
- Overproducing inflammatory compounds such as TMAO.
- Providing pathological signaling and associated increased inflammation, particularly in the brain.

Root Cause Candidate 3: NAD+

Research interest in NAD+ as a root cause of disease grows out of the field of anti-aging research and the discovery that NAD+ plays an important role in healthy mitochondrial function/energy production. NAD+ levels are known to drop with age, and this can contribute to many age-related illnesses.

At the time of this writing, Niagen and Elysium Basis, commercial NAD+ precursors based on nicotinamide riboside, are heavily marketed as anti-aging compounds. There is good evidence that supplementing with nicotinamide riboside raises NAD+ levels. Doing so is useful for improving mitochondrial function and energy production, which is particularly important as we age.

I take Niagen and think the science behind it is important. Nevertheless, I also think that marketing it as a silver bullet is short-sighted—a partial package that omits some really important information. You need to pay attention to NRF2 stimulation and glutathione levels as a complementary strategy to NAD+ repletion. Elysium Basis handles this by mixing pterostilbene (a polyphenol found in blueberries) with nicotinamide riboside to deal with both NRF2 stimulation and NAD+ repletion.

DNA Damage and NAD+: A Potential Feedforward Loop

One of the downstream impacts of increased oxidative stress is DNA damage. Just as your body has a stress response, it also has a DNA damage response to upregulate the DNA damage repair enzyme poly (ADP-ribose) polymerase (PARP). NAD+ is a raw material for PARP. Thus excess DNA damage can deplete NAD+ levels, resulting in metabolic dysregulation, mitochondrial dysfunction, and increased oxidative stress. Increased oxidative stress results in more DNA damage, and the cycle repeats as a potential feed-forward loop:

poly (ADP-ribose) polymerase (PARP) upregulation → DNA damage → upregulation, NAD+ depletion → mitochondrial dysfunction → increased oxidative stress.

Sugar Consumption and NAD+ Depletion

Over-consumption of processed carbohydrates and sugar activates the polyol pathway. The polyol pathway functions as safety valve to prevent the toxic build-up of glucose in blood and tissue by allowing the conversion of excess glucose to fructose. In this process, NAD+ is used by sorbitol dehydrogenase to convert sorbitol to fructose, contributing to NAD+ depletion.

NAD+: Key Takeaways

- Low NAD+ levels are a redox imbalance issue.
- NAD+ is a paradoxical compound since it is an oxidant, but lowering it puts your mitochondria in an inefficient mode that produces excess ROS, increasing oxidative stress. So raising this oxidant (NAD+) paradoxically lowers overall oxidative stress.
- This conundrum at least partially explains why redox imbalance is a more accurate term than oxidative stress. A NAD+ deficiency is technically "reductive stress" and a form of redox imbalance.
- NAD+ repletion via nicotinamide riboside supplementation represents one of the first commercial efforts to popularize a redox-focused therapy beyond the usual antioxidant vitamins. That is good news, but it needs to go further in explaining the science behind redox imbalance.
- NAD+ levels are depleted by a protein family called poly (ADP-ribose) polymerase (PARP) that is upregulated to handle DNA repair. DNA damage is caused by oxidative stress. What inhibits PARP? Plant Polyphenols, among other things.

Root Cause Candidate 4: Magnesium

Dr. Carolyn Dean's *The Magnesium Miracle* and similar books have done much to raise the profile of magnesium's role in maintaining health in the popular consciousness. The typical lead-in says that magnesium plays a role in more than three hundred biochemical processes as an enzyme cofactor, which it does. It goes on to explain how important magnesium is for heart health, diabetes, blood pressure, muscle function, bone health, and even things you might not expect, like thyroid function.

While there is general agreement that most Americans have some degree of magnesium deficiency, the cause is usually attributed to low-nutrient diets (not unreasonable) or falling levels of magnesium in the soil resulting in lower magnesium levels in food (maybe?). The stress/oxidative stress–magnesium deficiency connection is typically overlooked, and I believe that it holds the key to understanding the centrality of magnesium in health maintenance.

Important Concepts

- There is mounting evidence that stress and oxidative stress reduce intracellular magnesium levels. In restrained rat studies, which are designed to measure the impact of stress on said rats, one of the initial impacts is that serum magnesium actually *rises* as the stress causes a process called magnesium efflux, in which magnesium ions are pushed out of the cell via TRPV channels.
- Serum magnesium levels and intracellular magnesium levels are different, and intracellular levels are more important and more difficult to measure, which largely explains why magnesium is rarely measured and almost never accurately measured.
- Magnesium is a natural calcium channel blocker, meaning that diminished intracellular magnesium levels will raise intracellular calcium levels. Cellular calcium signaling primes pro-inflammatory cytokine release (via increased

substance P), and the resulting inflammatory stress has multiple downstream effects, such as raising blood pressure.[31] Magnesium also plays an important role in the heart's electrical function, so that a magnesium deficiency can cause heart arrhythmias and even sudden cardiac death.
- Certain classes of antibiotics (e.g., fluoroquinolones) lower magnesium levels and are associated with sudden cardiac death and muscle, tendon, and nerve issues.
- You cannot maintain a healthy antioxidant capacity if your magnesium levels are low, and supplementing with magnesium when it's low restores antioxidant capacity.
- You can test for low intracellular magnesium using a magnesium red blood cell (RBC) test, but this test is not commonly prescribed. A serum magnesium test is easier and more common, but less reliable since you can have normal or even high serum magnesium levels even when your intracellular levels are dangerously low.

Magnesium: Key Takeaways

Magnesium deficiency is closely linked to redox imbalance pathologies and treatment for the following reasons:
- I consider magnesium deficiency to be among the earliest and most common feedforward loops in redox imbalance, to the extent that if you are symptomatic in any way, you probably have some degree of magnesium deficiency.
- You cannot maintain healthy redox status with low intracellular magnesium status.
- Many researchers consider subclinical magnesium deficiency to be at epidemic levels.
- Low magnesium status is associated with every pathology of heart disease.
- Magnesium supplementation is beneficial in headaches, anxiety, and depression.

---

31 Nielsen, Forrest H. "Magnesium deficiency and increased inflammation: current perspectives." Journal of inflammation research vol. 11 25-34. 18 Jan. 2018, doi:10.2147/JIR.S136742

Root Cause Candidate 5: Inflammation

The November 2019 cover story in the monthly *AARP* magazine provocatively asked, "Could Decreasing Inflammation Be the Cure for Everything?" The subheading declared, "Managing your body's immune response is key to diseases of aging." That sounded a lot like the book I was writing, so I read the article with interest. There are countless books on inflammation and disease, anti-inflammatory diets, inflammation and aging. Still, this article made the boldest claim that I had run across for inflammation as a root cause of disease, and I wanted to evaluate how the claims held up. The verdict? Not bad. Here's why.

Recognition of inflammation as a part of the healing process after injury goes back to Hippocrates in the fifth century BCE. Inflammation goes hand-in-hand with the activation and work of the innate immune system. It's also tightly linked with oxidative stress, both because oxidative stress causes inflammation (think fire and burning) and because oxidative stress activates the immune system, stimulating the production of numerous inflammatory molecules, such as TNFα, IL-1β, IL-6, IL-17, and neutrophils. These inflammatory molecules produce more oxidative stress to kill pathogens. Generally speaking, where you find disease, you will find inflammation and oxidative stress, so inflammation is a good surrogate concept for oxidative stress. Nevertheless, it's really a symptom of damage and the disease process, whether physical, infectious, toxic, psychological, or nutritional—not the cause. Oxidative stress is the cause.

Inflammation: Key Takeaway

If there's something broadly understood as causing disease, there's an oxidative stress tie-in. Look for it. This is certainly true of inflammation.

Bottom Line: It's Still Redox Imbalance

All of these potential root causes play important roles in health and disease. Anti-aging research is generating some very exciting high-end therapeutics, and the emphasis on epigenetics is important. However, it's still redox imbalance that "scratches the DVD" and redox mechanisms mediating the adaptive stress response that confers stress resilience. Furthermore, top anti-aging compounds such as nicotinamide riboside, resveratrol, and pterostilbene are notable modulators of redox status.

The microbiome is also clearly very important in digestion, immune function, inflammation, and systemic regulation, directly linked to numerous diseases, including cancer, autoimmunity, pulmonary fibrosis, inflammatory bowel disease, etc. But while there are many bidirectional interactions between redox systems and the microbiome, the microbiome uses redox sensing and signaling mechanisms. Still, it is inarguably not the only user of those mechanisms. And when regulation of the microbiome and digestive tract goes off the rails, redox imbalance is involved, even when it's an upstream impact on the pancreas, gallbladder, or autonomic nervous system.

NAD+ research is exciting, but it's simply an integral part of our understanding of redox imbalance, specifically reductive stress and mitochondrial function/dysfunction.

As a glutathione cofactor, Magnesium is one of the key players in maintaining redox status and one of the early dysregulations growing out of psychological and oxidative stress of all kinds. Again, important but not the root cause.

Finally, inflammation is so inextricably tied to oxidative stress that I actually toyed with the idea of dropping the redox imbalance language entirely just to make things simpler for the masses. But in my experience, that kind of scientifically imprecise language always comes back to bite you eventually. Inflammation basically functions as a biomarker for oxidative stress, but it too is not the root cause.

The root cause of disease is (still) redox imbalance.

Chapter 6

Diagnosing Redox Imbalance

> *"Measurement is the first step that leads to control and eventually to improvement. If you can't measure something, you can't understand it. If you can't understand it, you can't control it. If you can't control it, you can't improve it."*
>
> —H. James Harrington

Earlier in the book, I referred to redox imbalance as the disease we don't measure, diagnose, or treat. It's no exaggeration to say that I wrote this book because I want the medical community to get on board to make this happen. However, to measure and diagnose a disease, you need biomarkers.

Biomarkers that are reliable, predictable, and broadly agreed upon are the foundation for both the definition and diagnosis of disease in Western medicine. For heart disease, it's been some variation of cholesterol and triglycerides for decades; for diabetes, it's HbA1C and fasting glucose; for liver disease, it's elevated liver enzymes.

In this chapter, we'll touch briefly on the history of our efforts to measure redox status, survey the growing body of strategies that have already been developed, and look at some promising new approaches with the potential to get us to the useful application of these ideas in a clinical setting.

Biomarkers For Oxidative Stress

For oxidative stress, there have been some intractable challenges standing in the way of adopting canonical biomarkers for clinical use. For starters, reactive species cannot be easily measured in bodily fluids because they have half-lives measured in nanoseconds to milliseconds. That means that redox biomarkers are at least one step removed from their root cause, typically the oxidative byproduct of an oxidant that no longer exists. Furthermore, there are many different kinds of redox reactions, so the biomarkers vary based on what is being oxidized where and by what reactive species. Finally, because redox status is compartmentalized to a sub-cellular level, taking redox biomarkers from bodily fluids (e.g., plasma) will measure generalized system-level redox imbalance, but not necessarily a location-specific redox imbalance.

Fifty Years of Measuring Redox Status

Despite the challenges, researchers have measured oxidative stress for years. In Helmut Sies' 1985 book "Oxidative Stress" attention was focused on the release of oxidized glutathione (GSSG) as an indicator of oxidative stress along with lipid oxidation. Because the initial concern was oxidative damage, the early emphasis focused on free radicals and the things being oxidized—lipids, DNA, proteins. Below is a partial timeline showing the evolution of oxidative stress-related biomarkers:
- The late 70s - 80s. Several studies connect the lipid peroxidation product malondialdehyde with peroxide 'oxidant stress.'
- 1987. Thiobarbituric acid reactive substances (TBARS) levels shown to rise in rats exposed to ethanol, while GSH and GSH/GSSG levels fell.[32]

---

32 Videla, L A et al. "Age-dependent changes in rat liver lipid peroxidation and glutathione content induced by acute ethanol ingestion." *Cell biochemistry and function* vol. 5,4 (1987): 273-80. doi:10.1002/cbf.290050406

- 1991. 8-hydroxy-2'-deoxyguanosine (oh8dG) and oh8Gua levels in urine proposed as a biomarker of DNA oxidative damage with particular relevance to cancer and aging.[33]
- 1993. The oxygen-radical absorbing capacity (ORAC) test described the total antioxidant capacity of a sample or food as a score. The test was adopted by the USDA and used to give an ORAC score to various foods. Over time, the test's validity was challenged, and the USDA ultimately withdrew it in 2012. The Ferric Reducing Ability of Plasma (FRAP) method for measuring total antioxidant capacity (TAC), introduced in the early 90s, is still used today.
- 1993. Advanced Glycation Endproducts (AGEs) are linked to stiffening of connective tissues and oxidative stress.
- 1993. Xanthine oxidase (XO), an enzymatic source of oxidative stress, is shown to be elevated in the serum of patients with inflammatory and autoimmune rheumatic disease. Treatment with corticosterone caused levels to return to normal.[34]
- 1994. F2-isoprostanes, formed when serum and LDL cholesterol are exposed to oxidants, proposed as a potential biomarker for oxidative stress.[35]
- 1996. Advanced Oxidation Protein Products (AOPPs) were identified as a biomarker of oxidative stress in uremia, a blood urea build-up in kidney disease.
- 2000. Protein carbonyls were proposed as a useful biomarker of oxidative stress.[36]

---

33 Shigenaga, M K, and B N Ames. "Assays for 8-hydroxy-2'-deoxyguanosine: a biomarker of in vivo oxidative DNA damage." *Free radical biology & medicine* vol. 10,3-4 (1991): 211-6. doi:10.1016/0891-5849(91)90078-h

34 Miesel, R, and M Zuber. "Elevated levels of xanthine oxidase in serum of patients with inflammatory and autoimmune rheumatic diseases." *Inflammation* vol. 17,5 (1993): 551-61. doi:10.1007/BF00914193

35 Lynch, S M et al. "Formation of non-cyclooxygenase-derived prostanoids (F2-isoprostanes) in plasma and low density lipoprotein exposed to oxidative stress in vitro." The Journal of clinical investigation vol. 93,3 (1994): 998-1004. doi:10.1172/JCI117107

36 Chevion, M et al. "Human studies related to protein oxidation: protein carbonyl content as a marker of damage." *Free radical research* vol. 33 Suppl (2000): S99-108.

- 2005. An automated test for determining Total Oxidant Status (TOS) of serum was introduced, and TOS was shown to be elevated in osteoarthritis patients. It is in current use as a research biomarker to this day.
- 2014. A new approach for measuring thiol/disulfide ratio is introduced.[37] At the time of publication, over 800 articles mostly show the clinical relevance of thiol/disulfide homeostasis in a wide range of diseases.
- 2016. Elevated Cystine/Glutathione ratio is shown to predict increased mortality in patients with coronary artery disease. The authors noted that this supported the notion that non-free radical oxidative processes were clinically important.[38]

Classifying the Strategies

Many approaches for measuring redox status have emerged with more on the horizon. Frankly, it can be a bit overwhelming. Indeed, others have noted that the proliferation of biomarkers is actually an impediment to the clinical application of the ideas behind redox imbalance/oxidative stress. Thus, it is useful to categorize the strategies as we think about how to best use the biomarkers at our disposal.

Measuring Ratios of Redox Couples

Your body has multiple interrelated systems for detoxifying free radicals and reactive species, and regulating redox status more broadly. These ratios can and have been measured in the primary redox couples:.

---

37 Erel, Ozcan, and Salim Neselioglu. "A novel and automated assay for thiol/disulphide homeostasis." *Clinical biochemistry* vol. 47,18 (2014): 326-32. doi:10.1016/j.clinbiochem.2014.09.026

38 Patel, Riyaz S et al. "Novel Biomarker of Oxidative Stress Is Associated With Risk of Death in Patients With Coronary Artery Disease." Circulation vol. 133,4 (2016): 361-9. doi:10.1161/CIRCULATIONAHA.115.019790

- Glutathione (GSH/GSSG ratio)
- Thioredoxin/Thioredoxin Reductase
- NADP/NADPH ratio
- Cys/CySS ratio
- NAD+/NADH ratio for reductive stress and metabolic function.

Measuring Redox Enzymes

Many studies have measured the level and activity of your body's antioxidant enzymes. Key enzymes for detoxifying reactive species include
- Superoxide dismutase
- Catalase
- Glutathione Peroxidase

Measuring Oxidative Byproducts

This is perhaps the most common strategy for measure oxidative stress, since the oxidative byproducts are much longer-lived than the oxidants that produced them and can be measured in bodily fluids. Examples include
- Malondialdehyde
- F2-isoprostanes
- Thiobarbituric acid reactive substances (TBARS)
- Advanced Oxidative Protein Products (AOPPs)

Measuring Redox Signaling Molecules

Elevated redox signaling molecule levels, particularly H_2O_2, can signal redox imbalance. Levels that are too low can indicate reductive stress.

Measuring Stress Load

One of the primary instruments available for measuring Stress Load is the Allostatic Load Index (ALI). While not perfect, ALI has been around for over two decades and has a track record for validity. The index is based on the following physiologic biomarkers:

- Systolic and diastolic blood pressure (autonomic dysregulation)
- Total cholesterol (cardiovascular risk, diet/lifestyle issues)
- High-density-lipoprotein (activity level)
- Glycosylated hemoglobin/HbA1c (metabolic health, diabetes)
- Waist-to-hip ratio (metabolic health, obesity),
- Dehydroepiandrosterone sulfate/DHEA-S (androgen, lowered under stress conditions)
- Epinephrine (stress hormone)
- Norepinephrine (stress hormone)
- Cortisol (stress hormone)

Other permutations of ALI include different biomarkers, such as heart rate (physical fitness, autonomic balance), albumin (nutritional status), and hsCRP (inflammation). Despite the heterogeneity of biomarker selection and analysis, measuring ALI has shown validity in workforce stress, pregnancy, racial/ethnic subgroups. Neutrophil-Lymphocyte Ratio (NLR), covered in more detail later in the chapter, could be considered an alternative approach to measuring stress load.

Measuring Nutritional Deficits

Accumulating evidence shows that nutritional deficits are commonly associated with redox imbalance, such as intracellular magnesium, vitamin D3, B12, folate, zinc, selenium, cysteine, thiamine, and niacin status.

Measuring the Electrical Reduction Potential of a Bodily Fluid (cOrp, sOrp)

This approach takes advantage of the electrochemical nature of oxidation-reduction reactions to measure the oxidation-reduction potential in a fluid, such as blood or semen. Aytu Biopharma produced devices that measure cOrp/sOrp but it appears they are no longer on the market.

Measuring Oxidative Stress-related MicroRNA (miRNA).

The role and function of an increasing number of miRNA are being catalogued and proposed as biomarkers. For example, upregulated miRNA-382 levels in kidney disease contribute to oxidative stress and renal fibrosis.[39]

Measuring Surrogates for Redox Imbalance

While measuring free radicals, oxidative byproducts, enzymes, signaling molecules, and redox couples get the most attention, the idea that there are surrogates that track with rising/falling redox status is a strategy with promise. Examples would include sympathetic/parasympathetic balance, inflammation, neutrophil/lymphocyte ratio (NLR), or heart rate variability (HRV).

Redox Biomarkers: From Bench to Bedside

As you can see, there is a large and growing array of strategies and biomarkers for oxidative stress. Each has its strengths and weaknesses and use cases. But while oxidative stress has been measured in research settings for decades (Bench), for biomarkers to be used in a clinical setting (Bedside), according to the World Health Organization, they must satisfy the following criteria:
1. They must be diagnostic for a specific disease.
2. They must have prognostic value, and
3. They must correlate with disease activity.

None of the existing redox biomarkers had met this criteria in large scale clinical trials until quite recently. Thus, despite accumulating evidence at a systems biology level that oxidative stress/redox imbalance caused or was a significant contributor to most diseases, the pathway to clinical acceptance was blocked. However, in the last five years, there have been several promising developments in the redox biomarker arena that promise to break down that barrier. Among them:

---

[39] Banerjee, Jaideep et al. "MicroRNA Regulation of Oxidative Stress." Oxidative medicine and cellular longevity vol. 2017 (2017): 2872156. doi:10.1155/2017/2872156

Cysteine-related Oxidative Stress Biomarkers

In the past decade, improvements to mass spectronomy technology have allowed researchers to measure cysteine, a sulfur amino acid, and its redox couple Cysteine/Cystine (Cys/CySS) with greater accuracy. These new abilities have led to an improved understanding of cysteine's role in maintaining and regulating cellular redox status, and more generally, how oxidative stress affects the body (e.g., mediating adaptive changes to metabolism through protein oxidation[40]). The significance for redox biomarkers has been that extracellular cysteine redox status directly impacts intracellular redox status, making serum cysteine-related biomarkers attractive candidates for measuring systemic oxidative stress. This has already had several manifestations; the first and most studied approach being the measuring of thiol-disulfide homeostasis.

Thiol/Disulfide Homeostasis

The ability to easily measure thiol/disulfide balance in a clinical setting got a significant boost in 2014 with a new automated process proposed by Erel and Neselioglu.[41] Since then, there's been an explosion of research and activity, applying this novel biomarker to a broad range of diseases and conditions. Thiols are the reduced forms of organosulfur compounds (e.g., cysteine and GSH), while disulfides are the oxidized forms (e.g., cystine, GSSG). Thus, thiol/disulfide balance is a biomarker that includes both oxidized and reduced components. Accumulating evidence indicates that the test is clinically relevant in a broad and growing range of diseases. I've thoroughly footnoted the list, which may seem like overkill to some, but I want you to scan the list and the footnotes to appreciate the breadth of diseases studied.

---

40 van der Reest, J., Lilla, S., Zheng, L. et al. "Proteome-wide analysis of cysteine oxidation reveals metabolic sensitivity to redox stress." Nat Commun 9, 1581 (2018), doi:10.1038/s41467-018-04003-3

41 Erel O, Neselioglu S. "A novel and automated assay for thiol/disulphide homeostasis." Clinical Biochemistry. 2014 Dec;47(18):326-332. DOI: 10.1016/j.clinbiochem.2014.09.026.

While the list contains a large number of small, observational studies, if borne out by larger clinical trials, measuring thiol-disulfide homeostasis could truly be a game-changer for redox biomarkers.

- Allergic rhinitis[42]
- Alzheimer's[43]
- Ankylosing spondylitis[44]
- Appendicitis[45]
- Arthritis[46]
- Behcet disease[47]
- Bipolar and unipolar depression[48]
- Bipolar disorder[49]
- Burns[50] (predicts severity and mortality)

---

42 Göker, Ayse E et al. "An Evaluation of Oxidative Stress With Thiol/Disulfide Homeostasis in Patients With Persistent Allergic Rhinitis." *Ear, nose, & throat journal*, 145561320926336. 20 Jul. 2020, doi:10.1177/0145561320926336

43 Gumusyayla, Sadiye et al. "A novel oxidative stress marker in patients with Alzheimer's disease: dynamic thiol-disulphide homeostasis." *Acta neuropsychiatrica* vol. 28,6 (2016): 315-320. doi:10.1017/neu.2016.13

44 Dogru, Atalay et al. "Thiol/disulfide homeostasis in patients with ankylosing spondylitis." *Bosnian journal of basic medical sciences* vol. 16,3 (2016): 187-92. doi:10.17305/bjbms.2016.1001

45 Ozyazici, Sefa et al. "A Novel Oxidative Stress Mediator in Acute Appendicitis: Thiol/Disulphide Homeostasis." *Mediators of inflammation* vol. 2016 (2016): 6761050. doi:10.1155/2016/6761050

46 Altinel Acoglu, Esma et al. "Changes in thiol/disulfide homeostasis in juvenile idiopathic arthritis." *Pediatrics international : official journal of the Japan Pediatric Society*vol. 60,6 (2018): 593-596. doi:10.1111/ped.13569

47 Balbaba, Mehmet et al. "Thiol/disulfide homeostasis in patients with ocular-active and ocular-inactive Behçet disease." *International ophthalmology*, 10.1007/s10792-020-01445-x. 1 Jun. 2020, doi:10.1007/s10792-020-01445-x

48 Erzin, Gamze et al. "Thiol/Disulfide Homeostasis in Bipolar and Unipolar Depression." *Clinical psychopharmacology and neuroscience : the official scientific journal of the Korean College of Neuropsychopharmacology* vol. 18,3 (2020): 395-401. doi:10.9758/cpn.2020.18.3.395

49 Cingi Yirün, Merve et al. "Thiol/disulphide homeostasis in manic episode and remission phases of bipolar disorder." *Nordic journal of psychiatry* vol. 72,8 (2018): 572-577. doi:10.1080/08039488.2018.1497200

50 Ergin Tuncay, Merve et al. "A remarkable point for evaluating the severity of burns: Thiol-disulfide profile." *Burns : journal of the International Society for Burn Injuries* vol. 46,4 (2020): 882-887. doi:10.1016/j.burns.2019.10.013

- Cancer[51,52,53]
- Cataract[54]
- Celiac disease[55]
- Childhood obesity[56]
- Colitis[57]
- Diabetes[58] (tracks with severity)
- Epilepsy[59]
- Erectile dysfunction[60]

---

51 Sezgin, Burak et al. "Assessment of thiol disulfide balance in early-stage endometrial cancer." *The journal of obstetrics and gynaecology research* vol. 46,7 (2020): 1140-1147. doi:10.1111/jog.14301

52 Sezgin, Burak et al. "Thiol-disulfide status of patients with cervical cancer." *The journal of obstetrics and gynaecology research*, 10.1111/jog.14480. 9 Sep. 2020, doi:10.1111/jog.14480

53 Eryilmaz, Mehmet Ali et al. "Thiol-disulfide homeostasis in breast cancer patients." *Journal of cancer research and therapeutics* vol. 15,5 (2019): 1062-1066. doi:10.4103/jcrt.JCRT_553_17

54 Elbay A, Ozer OF, Altinisik M, et al. A novel tool reflecting the role of oxidative stress in the cataracts: thiol/disulfide homeostasis. *Scand J Clin Lab Invest*. 2017;77(3):223-227. doi:10.1080/00365513.2017.1292539

55 Comba, Atakan et al. "Thiol-disulfide homeostasis in children with celiac disease." *Pediatrics international : official journal of the Japan Pediatric Society* vol. 62,8 (2020): 950-956. doi:10.1111/ped.14243

56 Mengen, Eda et al. "The Significance of Thiol/Disulfide Homeostasis and Ischemia-modified Albumin Levels in Assessing Oxidative Stress in Obese Children and Adolescents." *Journal of clinical research in pediatric endocrinology* vol. 12,1 (2020): 45-54. doi:10.4274/jcrpe.galenos.2019.2019.0039

57 Neselioglu, S et al. "The relationship between severity of ulcerative colitis and thiol-disulphide homeostasis." *Bratislavske lekarske listy* vol. 119,8 (2018): 498-502. doi:10.4149/BLL_2018_091

58 Gulpamuk, Bayram et al. "The significance of thiol/disulfide homeostasis and ischemia-modified albumin levels to assess the oxidative stress in patients with different stages of diabetes mellitus." *Scandinavian journal of clinical and laboratory investigation* vol. 78,1-2 (2018): 136-142.

59 Kösem, Arzu et al. "Evaluation of serum thiol-disulphide homeostasis parameters as oxidative stress markers in epilepsy patients." *Acta neurologica Belgica*, 10.1007/s13760-020-01410-6. 14 Jun. 2020, doi:10.1007/s13760-020-01410-6

60 Micoogullari, Uygar et al. "Thiol/Disulfide Homeostasis in Patients With Erectile Dysfunction." *The journal of sexual medicine*, S1743-6095(20)30760-8. 9 Aug. 2020, doi:10.1016/j.jsxm.2020.07.011

- Familial hypercholesterolemia[61]
- Gastritis (autoimmune)[62]
- Glaucoma[63]
- Heart disease[64]
- Heart failure[65]
- Hypertension[66]
- Hyperthyroidism (Graves' disease)[67]
- Hypothyroidism (Hashimoto's thyroiditis)[68]
- Inflammatory bowel disease (Crohn's disease, ulcerative colitis)[69]
- Jaundice (neonatal)[70]

---

61 Şimşek, Özgür et al. "Thiol/Disulfide Balance in Patients with Familial Hypercholesterolemia." *Cardiology research and practice* vol. 2018 9042461. 12 Jun. 2018, doi:10.1155/2018/9042461

62 Asfuroğlu Kalkan, Emra et al. "Thiol/disulfide homeostasis and ischemia modified albumin levels in autoimmune gastritis and their relations with gastric emptying." *Turkish journal of medical sciences* vol. 50,1 163-170. 13 Feb. 2020, doi:10.3906/sag-1902-17

63 Karakurt, Yucel et al. "Thiol-Disulfide Homeostasis and Serum Ischemia Modified Albumin Levels in Patients with Primary Open-Angle Glaucoma." *Current eye research* vol. 44,8 (2019): 896-900. doi:10.1080/02713683.2019.1594925

64 Altıparmak, Ibrahim Halil et al. "The relation of serum thiol levels and thiol/disulphide homeostasis with the severity of coronary artery disease." *Kardiologia polska* vol. 74,11 (2016): 1346-1353. doi:10.5603/KP.a2016.0085

65 Caliskan, Haci Mehmet et al. "Prognostic value of thiol/disulfide homeostasis in symptomatic patients with heart failure." *Archives of physiology and biochemistry*, 1-6. 4 Jun. 2020, doi:10.1080/13813455.2020.1773505

66 Ates, Ihsan et al. "Dynamic thiol/disulphide homeostasis in patients with newly diagnosed primary hypertension." *Journal of the American Society of Hypertension : JASH* vol. 10,2 (2016): 159-66. doi:10.1016/j.jash.2015.12.008

67 Agan, Veysel et al. "An Investigation of Oxidative Stress and Thiol/Disulphide Homeostasis in Graves' Disease." *Medicina (Kaunas, Lithuania)* vol. 55,6 275. 14 Jun. 2019, doi:10.3390/medicina55060275

68 Ates, Ihsan et al. "Dynamic thiol/disulfide homeostasis in patients with autoimmune subclinical hypothyroidism." *Endocrine research* vol. 41,4 (2016): 343-349. doi:10.3109/07435800.2016.1156124

69 Bourgonje, Arno R et al. "Serum Free Thiols Are Superior to Fecal Calprotectin in Reflecting Endoscopic Disease Activity in Inflammatory Bowel Disease." *Antioxidants (Basel, Switzerland)* vol. 8,9 351. 1 Sep. 2019, doi:10.3390/antiox8090351

70 Topal, Ismail et al. "Thiol-Disulfide Homeostasis, Serum Ferroxidase Activity, and Serum Ischemia Modified Albumin Levels in Neonatal Jaundice." *Fetal and pediatric pathology* vol. 38,2 (2019): 138-145. doi:10.1080/15513815.2018.1561772

- Kidney disease (nephropathy)[71]
- Macular degeneration, age-related[72]
- Migraine/headache[73]
- Multiple sclerosis[74]
- Otitis media (earache)[75]
- Parkinson's disease[76]
- Pancreatitis[77]
- Peripheral artery disease[78]
- Pneumonia[79]
- Polycystic ovary syndrome (PCOS)[80]

---

71 Eren, Mehmet Ali et al. "The evaluation of thiol/disulphide homeostasis in diabetic nephropathy." *Diabetes research and clinical practice* vol. 148 (2019): 249-253. doi:10.1016/j.diabres.2019.01.022

72 Elbay, Ahmet et al. "Comparison of serum thiol-disulphide homeostasis and total antioxidant-oxidant levels between exudative age-related macular degeneration patients and healthy subjects." *International ophthalmology* vol. 37,5 (2017): 1095-1101. doi:10.1007/s10792-016-0367-4

73 Kurt, Ayşegül Nese Citak et al. "Headache in children and dynamic thiol/disulfide balance evaluation with a new method." *Neurological sciences : official journal of the Italian Neurological Society and of the Italian Society of Clinical Neurophysiology* vol. 38,8 (2017): 1495-1499. doi:10.1007/s10072-017-3004-8

74 Vural, Gönül et al. "Relationship between thiol-disulphide homeostasis and visual evoked potentials in patients with multiple sclerosis." *Neurological sciences : official journal of the Italian Neurological Society and of the Italian Society of Clinical Neurophysiology* vol. 40,2 (2019): 385-391. doi:10.1007/s10072-018-3660-3

75 Şimşek, Eda et al. "Is otitis media with effusion associated with oxidative stress? Evaluation of thiol/disulfide homeostasis." *American journal of otolaryngology* vol. 40,2 (2019): 164-167. doi:10.1016/j.amjoto.2018.12.012

76 Vural, Gonul et al. "Impairment of dynamic thiol-disulphide homeostasis in patients with idiopathic Parkinson's disease and its relationship with clinical stage of disease." *Clinical neurology and neurosurgery* vol. 153 (2017): 50-55. doi:10.1016/j.clineuro.2016.12.009

77 Uyanıkoğlu, Ahmet et al. "Impaired thiol/disulfide homeostasis in patients with mild acute pancreatitis." *The Turkish journal of gastroenterology : the official journal of Turkish Society of Gastroenterology* vol. 30,10 (2019): 899-902. doi:10.5152/tjg.2019.18775

78 Korkmaz, Ufuk Turan Kursat et al. "Dynamic thiol/disulphide homeostasis metrics as a risk factor for peripheral arterial disease." *Vascular*, 1708538120947245. 9 Aug. 2020, doi:10.1177/1708538120947245

79 Parlak, Ebru S et al. "Evaluation of dynamic thiol/disulfide redox state in community-acquired pneumonia." *Saudi medical journal* vol. 39,5 (2018): 495-499. doi:10.15537/smj.2018.5.22111

80 Tola, Esra Nur et al. "The Role of Follicular Fluid Thiol/Disulphide Homeostasis in Polycystic Ovary Syndrome." *Balkan medical journal* vol. 35,4 (2018): 306-310. doi:10.4274/balkanmedj.2017.1140

Diagnosing Redox Imbalance

- Preeclampsia[81]
- Psoriasis[82]
- Recurrent pregnancy loss[83]
- Schizophrenia[84]
- Sepsis[85]
- Sleep apnea[86]
- Stroke[87]
- Tinnitus[88]
- Trauma (gunshot wounds)[89]
- Urticaria (rash)[90]

---

81 Onat, Taylan et al. "The relationship between oxidative stress and preeclampsia. The serum ischemia-modified albumin levels and thiol/disulfide homeostasis." *Turkish journal of obstetrics and gynecology* vol. 17,2 (2020): 102-107. doi:10.4274/tjod.galenos.2020.23682

82 Aksoy, Mustafa, and Adnan Kirmit. "Thiol/disulphide balance in patients with psoriasis." *Postepy dermatologii i alergologii vol.* 37,1 (2020): 52-55. doi:10.5114/ada.2018.77767

83 Erkenekli, Kudret et al. "Thiol/disulfide homeostasis in patients with idiopathic recurrent pregnancy loss assessed by a novel assay: Report of a preliminary study." *The journal of obstetrics and gynaecology research* vol. 42,2 (2016): 136-41. doi:10.1111/jog.12860

84 Ünal, Kübranur et al. "Thiol/disulphide homeostasis in schizophrenia patients with positive symptoms." *Nordic journal of psychiatry* vol. 72,4 (2018): 281-284. doi:10.1080/08039488.2018.1441906

85 Yildiz, Hamit. "Thiol/disulfide homeostasis in intensive care unit patients with sepsis and septic shock." *Turkish journal of medical sciences*, vol. 50,4 811–816. 31 Mar. 2020, doi:10.3906/sag-1905-148

86 Sengoren Dikis, Ozlem et al. "The relationship of thiol/disulfide homeostasis in the etiology of patients with obstructive sleep apnea: a case-control study." *The aging male : the official journal of the International Society for the Study of the Aging Male*, 1-8. 3 Apr. 2019, doi:10.1080/13685538.2019.1573890

87 Bektas, Hesna et al. "Dynamic thiol-disulfide homeostasis in acute ischemic stroke patients." *Acta neurologica Belgica* vol. 116,4 (2016): 489-494. doi:10.1007/s13760-016-0598-1

88 Celik, Mustafa, and İsmail Koyuncu. "A Comprehensive Study of Oxidative Stress in Tinnitus Patients." *Indian journal of otolaryngology and head and neck surgery : official publication of the Association of Otolaryngologists of India* vol. 70,4 (2018): 521-526. doi:10.1007/s12070-018-1464-7

89 Buyukaslan, Hasan et al. "Serum thiol levels and thiol/disulphide homeostasis in gunshot injuries." *European journal of trauma and emergency surgery : official publication of the European Trauma Society* vol. 45,1 (2019): 167-174. doi:10.1007/s00068-017-0900-9

90 Akdag, Songul et al. "Assessment of thiol/disulphide homoeostasis and ischaemia-modified albumin and their relationship with disease severity in children with chronic urticaria." *Cutaneous and ocular toxicology* vol. 39,3 (2020): 269-273. doi:10.1080/15569527.2020.1790589

- Vertigo[91]
- Warts[92]

Other Cysteine-related Biomarkers

A second significant milestone occurred in 2016, with a study of 1,411 patients undergoing cardiac angiography showing that elevated serum cystine/glutathione ratio predicted mortality in patients with coronary artery disease.[93] The biomarker measures oxidative burden (via cystine) and resilience to that oxidative burden (via glutathione/GSH) in serum. The redox research community regarded the knowledge that this serum biomarker was highly-predictive of death in a clinical setting as a watershed moment for redox biomarkers.

While these are promising developments, and I expect some manifestation of cysteine-related biomarkers to gain clinical acceptance, the pathway to broad usage will likely be measured in years, as more clinical trials and reviews validate the approaches.

Neutrophil-Lymphocyte Ratio (NLR) as a Biomarker for Redox Imbalance

For many years, doctors have used complete blood count (CBC) tests to screen for various pathologies such as anemia, infections, and leukemia. The test is cheap (about $30 - $50), reliable, and readily available. You probably already have multiple CBC tests in your health record. More recently, researchers have created synthetic biomarkers from CBC test components that track with oxidative stress and inflammation.

---

91 Şahin, Ethem et al. "Oxidative Status in Patients with Benign Paroxysmal Positional Vertigo." *The journal of international advanced otology* vol. 14,2 (2018): 299-303. doi:10.5152/iao.2018.4756

92 Erturan, I et al. "Evaluation of oxidative stress in patients with recalcitrant warts." *Journal of the European Academy of Dermatology and Venereology : JEADV* vol. 33,10 (2019): 1952-1957. doi:10.1111/jdv.15746

93 Patel, Riyaz S et al. "Novel Biomarker of Oxidative Stress Is Associated With Risk of Death in Patients With Coronary Artery Disease." *Circulation* vol. 133,4 (2016): 361-9. doi:10.1161/CIRCULATIONAHA.115.019790

Synthetic biomarkers simply use more than one biomarker, typically expressed as a ratio, to create something more useful and predictive than the individual markers alone. For example, a waist/height ratio is considered a superior biomarker for obesity than BMI, with a 1:2 ratio being the standard cut-off point for central obesity.

Researchers have looked at a variety of these synthetic biomarkers, and the ones with a degree of predictive value include

- Monocyte/lymphocyte ratio (MLR).
- Neutrophil/lymphocyte ratio (NLR).
- Monocyte/HDL ratio (MHR).
- Platelet/lymphocyte ratio (PLR).
- Systemic immune-inflammation index (SII), calculated with the formula $SII = (P \times N)/L$, where P, N, and L refer to peripheral platelet, neutrophil, and lymphocyte counts, respectively.

Of the above biomarkers, neutrophil/lymphocyte ratio has had by far the most research attention, with nearly 5,000 published articles on PubMed. While we cannot begin to cover all the learnings from these studies, certain patterns emerge when NLR is elevated:

- It tracks with disease severity in conditions such as appendicitis[94] and COVID-19.[95]
- It predicts worse outcomes. For example, an NLR ≥ 4 was associated with worse outcomes in inflammatory breast cancer.[96]

---

[94] Ozkan, Atakan et al. "The importance of laboratory tests and Body Mass Index in the diagnosis of acute appendicitis." *Polski przeglad chirurgiczny* vol. 92,5 (2020): 1-5.

[95] Asan, Ali et al. "Do initial hematologic indices predict the severity of COVID-19 patients?." *Turkish journal of medical sciences*, 10.3906/sag-2007-97. 2 Oct. 2020, doi:10.3906/sag-2007-97

[96] Van Berckelaer, C et al. "A high neutrophil-lymphocyte ratio and platelet-lymphocyte ratio are associated with a worse outcome in inflammatory breast cancer." *Breast (Edinburgh, Scotland)* vol. 53 (2020): 212-220. doi:10.1016/j.breast.2020.08.006

- It predicts mortality in conditions such as chronic kidney disease,[97] COPD,[98] sepsis,[99] and COVID-19.[100]
- It predicts comorbidities. An NLR ≥ 5 predicted liver damage in severe COVID-19 cases.[101]
- It predicts the occurrence of certain health issues, such as pregnancy loss,[102] and erectile dysfunction (NLR > 3)[103]
- It predicts recurrence in certain cancers, such as colon cancer.[104]

The Case for NLR as a Redox Biomarker

Though it is based solely on white blood cell components, NLR is typically framed as a biomarker for inflammation. However, more recently, several studies have noted that NLR can be thought of in ways that make it very interesting as an oxidative stress biomarker.

---

97 Ao, Guangyu et al. "Association of neutrophil-to-lymphocyte ratio and risk of cardiovascular or all-cause mortality in chronic kidney disease: a meta-analysis." *Clinical and experimental nephrology*, 10.1007/s10157-020-01975-9. 6 Oct. 2020, doi:10.1007/s10157-020-01975-9

98 Guo, Rui et al. "The predictive value of neutrophil-to-lymphocyte ratio for chronic obstructive pulmonary disease: a systematic review and meta-analysis." *Expert review of respiratory medicine* vol. 14,9 (2020): 929-936. doi:10.1080/17476348.2020.1776613

99 Huang, Zhiwei et al. "Prognostic value of neutrophil-to-lymphocyte ratio in sepsis: A meta-analysis." *The American journal of emergency medicine* vol. 38,3 (2020): 641-647. doi:10.1016/j.ajem.2019.10.023a

100 Wang, Shijie et al. "Neutrophil-to-lymphocyte ratio at admission is an independent risk factors for the severity and mortality in patients with coronavirus disease 2019." *The Journal of infection*, S0163-4453(20)30630-7. 23 Sep. 2020, doi:10.1016/j.jinf.2020.09.022

101 Wang, Ming et al. "Clinical characteristics and risk factors of liver injury in COVID-19: a retrospective cohort study from Wuhan, China." *Hepatology international*, 10.1007/s12072-020-10075-5. 7 Oct. 2020, doi:10.1007/s12072-020-10075-5

102 Bas, Funda Yildirim et al. "The role of complete blood inflammation markers in the prediction of spontaneous abortion." *Pakistan journal of medical sciences* vol. 34,6 (2018): 1381-1385. doi:10.12669/pjms.346.15939

103 Ventimiglia, E et al. "The role of neutrophil-to-lymphocyte ratio in men with erectile dysfunction-preliminary findings of a real-life cross-sectional study." *Andrology* vol. 6,4 (2018): 559-563. doi:10.1111/andr.12489

104 Balde, Alpha I et al. "Propensity score analysis of recurrence for neutrophil-to-lymphocyte ratio in colorectal cancer." *The Journal of surgical research* vol. 219 (2017): 244-252. doi:10.1016/j.jss.2017.05.109

NLR as a Biomarker of Physiologic Stress

In a body under increased physiologic stress, neutrophil counts go up, and lymphocyte counts go down. The technical names for this are neutrophilia and lymphopenia. Oxidative stress is linked to both phenomena. Thus, under extreme physiologic stress, we can expect the NLR to rise far beyond the typical 1-2 range, indicating the severity of the stress burden. A man in his late 60s who experienced multiple heart attacks recorded NLR values over 30 in the midst of his health crisis. Two years later, his NLR values had returned to well below 2. Physiologic stress invokes the body's stress response with associated increased ROS production and oxidative stress.

NLR as a Biomarker of Immune System Activation/Dysregulation

Neutrophils are "first on the scene" innate immune system responders to damage and pathogen activity. So when they, and by extension NLR, are high, the immune system is activated and generating oxidative stress and inflammation via the neutrophil "respiratory burst" and later through the recruitment of other inflammatory mediators—chemokines, cytokines, IL1-B, IL-6, TNF-a, etc.

NLR as a Biomarker of Stress Resilience

One author noting the wide range of diseases where NLR is predictive of onset, severity, and worse outcomes, wryly remarked that a biomarker that predicts every disease predicts no disease. Research into NLR and COVID-19 showed NLR functioning as a biomarker of stress resilience, making it useful for risk stratification of newly hospitalized patients. Knowing who is likely to advance to severe disease has treatment ramifications that can ultimately improve outcomes.

NLR as a Biomarker of Oxidative Stress

Several studies have shown NLR closely correlating with oxidative stress biomarkers, the most recent being a fascinating study on astronauts and low-gravity situations. Astronauts and rodents exposed to microgravity in space flight both showed elevated NLR levels. In the study, rats exposed to simulated microgravity showed elevated oxidative stress biomarkers and increased neutrophil counts, which returned to normal with antioxidant supplementation. The study concluded that "...modifying mechanisms involved in ROS-driven inflammation may provide a promising avenue to limit chronic inflammation and maintain homeostatic immunity during long-duration missions."[105]

While not explicitly an oxidative stress biomarker, NLR's breadth of evidence showing prognostic ability and potential utility in clinical settings, ubiquity, simplicity, low-cost and strong correlation with physiologic stress and oxidative stress biomarkers make it a highly attractive "good enough" biomarker for screening large populations for risks associated with redox imbalance.

A Classification Framework for Standard Redox Biomarkers

While individual redox biomarkers had failed to live up to clinical expectations, researchers increasingly recognized that leveraging multiple redox biomarkers was a promising strategy to overcome the limitations of any single biomarker. In a 2020 article, Pietro Ghezzi proposed a classification framework for redox biomarkers made of 5 'types' that I believe helps us make better use of existing redox biomarkers.[106] They are:

- **Type O**. Direct measurement of ROS. This has been considered impractical given the short half-life of reactive species, but there are recent papers detailing strategies to do it. Nevertheless, I think it will be years before we see

---

105 Paul, Amber M et al. "Neutrophil-to-Lymphocyte Ratio: A Biomarker to Monitor the Immune Status of Astronauts." *Frontiers in immunology* vol. 11 564950. 2 Nov. 2020, doi:10.3389/fimmu.2020.564950

106 Ghezzi, Pietro. "Environmental risk factors and their footprints in vivo - A proposal for the classification of oxidative stress biomarkers." *Redox biology* vol. 34 (2020): 101442. doi:10.1016/j.redox.2020.101442

this approach in broad use, hence the use of zero in the name.
- **Type 1.** Biomarkers of oxidative stress. Ghezzi surveys the literature and comes up with a list of oxidation byproducts that includes
  - Oxidized proteins (Protein carbonyls, IMA)
  - Oxidized lipids (MDA, isoprostanes, HNE, oxLDL)
  - Oxidized DNA (8-OH-dG)
- **Type 2.** Biomarkers indicating ROS-generating enzymes have been activated. This is a short list that includes uric acid, allantoin, and HOCl.
- **Type 3.** Biomarkers measuring factors that determine the susceptibility to oxidative damage.
  - Superoxide dismutase (SOD)
  - Catalase (CAT)
  - Glutathione Peroxidase (GPX)
  - Paraoxonase 1 (PON1)
  - Xanthine oxidase (XO)
  - NADP Oxidase (NOX)
  - Dual Oxidase (DUOX)
  - Vitamins C and E
  - Total Antioxidant Status/Capacity (TAS/TAC)
  - Bilirubin
- **Type 4.** Genetic factors and mutations affecting enzymes associated with ROS production and detoxification. These can be thought of as host-susceptibility factors and would include Down Syndrome, where a duplicate chromosome 21 causes lifelong overproduction of SOD.

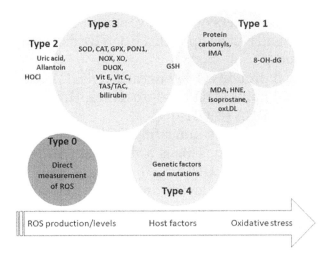

Figure X. Ghezzi's Classification Framework for Oxidative Stress Biomarkers. Note that the Types flow from left to right, implying sequence and progression, from ROS production/overproduction to adaptive responses and host factors to oxidative stress and oxidative damage. Used with permission.

In addition to acknowledging and classifying the different roles various biomarkers play in redox regulation/dysregulation, Ghezzi uses the framework to show sequence and progression over time and host factors that help shape pathological outcomes. This approach helps guide our thinking about groupings of existing biomarkers that might be deployed in ways that have greater prognostic value.

The above three developments (the rise of cysteine-related OS biomarkers, the rise of NLR and blood-based synthetic biomarkers, and a framework for leveraging multiple OS biomarkers) form the foundation I predict will be a workable clinical biomarker strategy to diagnose oxidative stress for both disease prevention and treatment. Because the clinical validation process is slow and methodical, you will see these strategies appear in functional medicine and alternative medicine practices before being approved for use by your local MD.

Biomarkers of Oxidative Stress and Inflammation: Key Takeaways

Clinical application of the ideas behind redox imbalance cannot happen without agreed-upon biomarkers, even imperfect ones. Thus far, we've detailed the beginnings of what I think is a workable biomarker strategy for oxidative stress, the key takeaways being:

1. **It's incredibly useful to have common biomarkers.** There's no doubt in my mind that increasing acceptance of biomarkers such as NLR and thiol/disulfide ratio as clinically useful will create a virtuous cycle where more researchers will find new uses and new therapies that in turn draw in more researchers and clinicians to build on that success.
2. **NLR is a solid candidate for the "good enough" oxidative stress biomarker** for population-level screening. As a part of the Complete Blood Count, it's cheap, easy, ubiquitous, consistent, well-understood by medical professionals, and remarkably predictive as a biomarker in a broad range of diseases. Because neutrophils rise with stress while lymphocytes fall, the ratio is very effective for measuring physiological stress that tracks well with oxidative stress biomarkers.
3. **Thiol/disulfide testing should be understood as a biomarker for oxidative stress and antioxidant capacity**, with high thiol levels indicating an abundance of capacity to reduce oxidants and disulfide measuring the amount of oxidized thiols.
4. **Low native and total thiol levels are indicative of disease and track with disease severity.** This outcome occurred in study after study and validates my original hypothesis that redox imbalance causes disease in a way I could barely have imagined. It happened in acute conditions like trauma (gunshot wounds), in autoimmune diseases, cancers, cardiovascular diseases, lung, kidney, liver diseases, skin conditions, pregnancy and infertility,

depression, neurodegenerative diseases, even warts! The only time it didn't was at the onset of a condition such as head injury, where thiols rose as a protective response against the trauma. A second scenario occurred when the redox imbalance was localized to the extent that a general blood test didn't measure a difference between patients and controls, as was the case in PCOS. A second study measuring localized follicular fluid did indeed find a thiol/disulfide imbalance, indicating oxidative stress.

5. **Higher thiol levels were protective.** In some instances, researchers treated the patients, retested, and found the thiol/disulfide imbalance resolved or improved.
6. **Higher disulfide levels were typically associated with disease.** While not quite as prevalent as the low-thiol/disease connection, high disulfide levels were routinely associated with disease, disease progression, and severity.
7. **We'll be mining this strategy for years.** There are still diseases that haven't been studied for the relevance of these biomarkers. Furthermore, proving causality, finding underlying modes of action, and testing the efficacy of redox therapies will take years.
8. **We already know how to modulate the redox imbalance associated with disrupted thiol/disulfide status and dysregulated immune function.** If anything, there are too many strategies, and thus we will spend years debating which ones work the best, are the cheapest, most reliable, and safest, have the fewest side effects, etc.

Biomarkers for Reductive Stress

There were many times while writing this book that I cursed the existence of reductive stress. Everything would be so much simpler and easier to explain. We'd talk about oxidative stress instead of redox imbalance. We'd treat oxidative stress with antioxidants, and it would all be good. The problem is, we've already gone down that road, and it didn't work out very well. Reductive stress is real. It has far less visibility than oxidative stress, and there's nothing quite analogous to the thiol/disulfide test for reductive stress. Still, it has to be factored in as you treat oxidative stress. Reductive stress is the pendulum swing you are trying to avoid when treating oxidative stress and pathological redox signaling. In redox balance, it is the Yin to oxidative stress's Yang.

NAD+/NADH Ratio: The Superstar Biomarker for Reductive Stress

Thanks to a growing anti-aging industry, NAD+ has been advertised relentlessly, and research indicates it's more than just a fad. NAD+ is an oxidant, and the NAD+/NADH pool needs to be maintained in an oxidized state for a healthy metabolism. Researchers have measured the NAD+/NADH ratio for years, and there are commercial testing kits available, though definitely not consumer-grade, point-of-care tests. From the research, we know with increasing confidence that NAD+ levels fall with age and ill health.[107] And we know that there is therapeutic benefit for metabolic health in raising NAD+ levels when they are low.

---

107 Johnson, Sean, and Shin-Ichiro Imai. "NAD + biosynthesis, aging, and disease." *F1000Research* vol. 7 132. 1 Feb. 2018, doi:10.12688/f1000research.12120.1

Reductive Imbalance in Other Redox Couples

While at this point vastly less studied, reductive imbalances in other redox couples including NADP/NADPH and GSH/GSSG are beginning to get research attention, particularly in energy production, cellular redox homeostasis and redox signaling.[108] It stands to reason that as clinical interest in bolstering and modulating redox status increases that reductive stress and the need to measure it would also receive additional research attention.

Redox Health Biomarkers for Patients

For patients/health consumers, though it may sound flippant, if you're symptomatic, you are most likely in a state of redox imbalance. This turns out to be both useful and empowering since we as patients often know what the stressors are and can develop useful strategies that resolve or improve the issue and keep us out of the medical system. Symptoms become our biomarkers, and we share them with our doctors to hasten the diagnosis. Some manifestation of this process has been going on since the dawn of civilization. What's relatively new is the simple, low-cost ability for health consumers to amass a trove of clinically relevant health data. While not directly related to redox status, these data and biomarkers can tip us off that redox imbalance is present and affecting the balance of our bodily systems.

Consumer-Accessible Biomarkers for Downstream Systemic Dysregulation

Chronic redox imbalance can rapidly result in dysregulation of multiple bodily systems. While the core redox therapies

---

108 Xiao, Wusheng, and Joseph Loscalzo. "Metabolic Responses to Reductive Stress." *Antioxidants & redox signaling* vol. 32,18 (2020): 1330-1347. doi:10.1089/ars.2019.7803

are stress reduction/mitigation, bolstering stress resilience with low-level eustressors such as exercise, calorie restriction, plant-based diets, and intermittent fasting, it is still necessary and useful to understand the downstream dysregulations. In many instances, systemic dysregulation of the autonomic nervous system, immune system, metabolism, HPA axis, gut microbiome, and gut and vascular barriers is participating in self-sustaining, pro-oxidant loops that need to be addressed directly, not just by mitigating the stressors and expecting the symptoms to resolve on their own.

Sympathetic/Parasympathetic Imbalance and the Autonomic Nervous System

Hyperactivation of the sympathetic nervous system is epidemic in our high-stress society. The availability of increasingly sophisticated fitness trackers and wearables makes it easy to track biomarkers predictive of sympathetic/parasympathetic imbalance such as resting heart rate and heart rate variability (HRV). Combined with an at-home, upper-arm blood pressure cuff (typically under $50), health consumers have potent tools for understanding these imbalances.

Vagus nerve stimulation has also emerged as a useful therapeutic approach for restoring balance to the autonomic nervous system. While surgical implantation of vagus nerve stimulators is an option, most people can achieve significant benefit through non-invasive vagus nerve stimulation approaches such as deep breathing exercises, yoga, meditation/prayer, qigong routines, acupressure, and massage.

Redox Biomarkers: Future Directions

While I expect a maturing and increasingly nuanced understanding of the biomarkers presented in this chapter, I'm in no way convinced that additional breakthroughs are out of reach. Below is just a sampling of the emerging fields destined to impact measurement of redox imbalance.

Metabolomic Screening

The new field of metabolomics uses high-throughput screening to identify new candidate biomarkers and potentially screen for disease susceptibility, initiation, and progression. The field is still in its infancy, but as costs fall and strategies improve, this looks like a promising direction.

MicroRNA Biomarkers and Therapeutics

Work has already begun on identifying microRNAs responsible for epigenetic regulation of oxidative stress and antioxidant protection in diverse diseases, including cardiovascular disease, cancer, diabetes, aging, heart attack, liver and kidney disease.[109] While mainstream use of microRNA therapeutics is likely years out, specific microRNA involved in pathology and protection are being identified and therapeutic potential proposed. At the very minimum, this research is giving us a clearer and more granular picture of how certain redox-related functions work

Mobile Health/Continuous Monitoring

At this writing, we are seeing consumer devices grow increasingly sophisticated as health monitoring devices. The Apple Watch provides monitoring of an expanding array of targeted health biomarkers—currently including blood oxygen saturation, VO_2 max, sleep tracking, heart rate variability (each morning), heart rate (continuous), and electrocardiogram (on demand).

As time and technology advance, one can reasonably predict that new low-cost sensors will expand the breadth, accuracy, and sophistication possible. Fitbit's latest watch offers an electrodermal activity sensor to measure stress.

---

[109] Banerjee, Jaideep et al. "MicroRNA Regulation of Oxidative Stress." Oxidative medicine and cellular longevity vol. 2017 (2017): 2872156. doi:10.1155/2017/2872156

Other devices offer sleep tracking, blood pressure monitoring, and even continuous glucose monitoring. Bluetooth can connect medical devices such as spirometers to smartphones and smartwatches to store medical data in applications such as Apple Health and Google Fit.

The earlier discussion on blood component biomarkers points to a broad range of opportunities for more sophisticated analysis of raw health data to inform both consumers and healthcare professionals of elevated risks for adverse health events, such as cancer, heart disease, and stroke. Labs such as Quest Diagnostics already integrate with Apple Health, so this prospect is more about the legal and regulatory ramifications of providing the information rather than a technological challenge.

The list of clinically relevant biomarkers and data that an average consumer can gather with a smartwatch and a relatively small investment in other health testing peripherals is long and growing longer:

- Waist/height ratio > 1:2. Your device knows you're overweight.
- Resting heart rate (RHR) above 70. You have some degree of autonomic dysregulation. Higher RHR is a risk factor for mortality.
- Low HRV values. Combined with age and gender, HRV can be presented in table form to assess relative cardiovascular fitness, sympathetic/parasympathetic balance in the autonomic nervous system.
- Blood pressure over 140/90. Dysregulation of the autonomic nervous system and renin-angiotensin-aldosterone system, electrolyte imbalance, and probable lowered nutritional status.
- HbA1C > 6. Pre-diabetes, diabetes, mitochondrial dysfunction, inflammation.
- Elevated Neutrophil-Lymphocyte ratio and Sii. Elevated systemic inflammation and oxidative stress, dysregulated immune system, increased cancer risk, increased risk for

adverse health events, lowered stress resilience.
- Overnight blood oxygen level < 90 percent. Possible sleep apnea. Increased risk for cardiovascular disease, diabetes, and sudden death. There is still controversy over the accuracy of spO2 wrist readings at the time of publication, though it's reasonable to assume these will continue to improve over time.
- The Prognostic Nutritional Index (PNI), a clinically-relevant biomarker for nutritional status, can be calculated based on the formula $10 \times$ serum albumin (g/dL)) + ($0.005 \times$ total lymphocyte count. Though non-specific, PNI is easy to calculate and could allow your mobile device to recommend more specific testing of nutritional status.
- VO_2 max, age, and gender combined give us a window into relative lung health and aerobic fitness. The Apple Watch and other fitness trackers provide a relative or predicted VO_2 max score, which though less sophisticated than a hospital stress test, is nonetheless considered accurate enough to be useful.

While some of this data currently has to be either manually entered or uploaded from lab tests, combined with genomic data from sites like 23andMe, the emerging picture is a world where your health status can be monitored in near real-time, with analysis that is practically unlimited in its sophistication. That utopian health vision needs to be tempered by the security and privacy challenges we currently face. Yet, it's hard to imagine not moving quickly in this direction, given the prospect of potentially life-saving health information delivered to your smartphone at minimal cost.

.

Chapter 7

Redox Self-care: Prevention Through Resilience

> *"What doesn't kill you, makes you stronger"*
> — *Friedrich Nietzsche*

The journey to health and wellness begins with holistic self-care. Its goal is the resilience that prevents disease, overcomes adversity and loss, and helps you maximize your potential as a human being. Success, happiness, and fulfillment are byproducts. This chapter wasn't in the original manuscript. Still, as I reflected on the role of redox systems in adaptation to stress and specifically the concepts of eustressors and hormesis, I was struck that the strongest argument for adopting a redox-centric view of health and disease was here in the sphere of self-care. This is partly due to the paucity of FDA-approved pharmaceuticals specifically to treat redox imbalance and the medical establishment's non-recognition of the role redox imbalance plays in health and disease. In some ways, that turns out to be a plus. How so? You are in charge of your health. It's always been true, even though, at times, it may feel like you're a passive participant. The point of this book and this chapter specifically is to empower you with ideas, information, and practical steps to maintain and improve your health and well-being.

Self-care and Resilience Habits

At the core of redox self-care is a collection of what I refer to as "resilience habits." For our purposes, resilience habits are either:

1. **Eustressors**—where an acute stressor, like exercise or eating leafy greens, invokes an adaptive stress response and epigenetic changes that make the body more resilient to future stress.
2. **Destressors**—where an activity or practice decreases stress burden to a point and a duration that allows for recovery from chronic stress, restoration of stress resilience, and a return to regulatory balance of downstream bodily systems. Destressors include sleep, naps, sabbath, vacation, play, sex, prayer, meditation, forgiveness, laughter, social connection, and other healthy practices and coping strategies that may be specific just to you.

The key tenet behind resilience habits is that resilience can be lost, resulting in increased vulnerability to illness, injury, and disease symptoms such as anxiety, depression, colds, headaches, pain, acid reflux, and even cancer. But resilience can also be recovered and enhanced through resilience habits that reduce symptom frequency and severity, prevent disease or shorten its duration and severity. I cannot overstate how important it is for you to understand and believe that resilience can be recovered and enhanced. Prevention through resilience is our goal. Let's get started.

The Evolution of Self-care

The idea of self-care is certainly not new, though its original medical meaning was almost entirely about convalescence and moving from total dependence to self-care. Hospitals of the mid-20th century had "self-care wards," which were contrasted with "intensive-care wards," and housed people who had recovered to the point that they could function somewhat independently, but not to the point that they could be released. Self-care was also tightly linked to self-management of your diagnosed condition, e.g., can you self-administer your diabetes meds or injections? However, by the end of the 20th century, societal shifts such as the burgeoning self-help movement, popular psychology, and increasing interest in eastern spiritual practices helped morph self-care into something much closer to the current understanding, which includes a greater emphasis on mental health and emotional wellbeing, along with clear linkage to a holistic understanding of wellness. Depending on who you ask, this holistic approach to wellness has somewhere between 5 and 10 components, including

1. Physical
2. Emotional
3. Social
4. Spiritual
5. Intellectual/Mental

with others adding:

6. Vocational/Occupational
7. Nutritional
8. Financial
9. Environmental
10. Creative

I would affirm each of these components' roles, with the observation that each can play a role in eustress or distress, and each has resilience practices that can contribute to physical and emotional resilience.

Why Redox Self-care?

As I write this chapter, I am keenly aware that I am not the first to write about self-care, holistic wellness, or even the health-inducing practices that I classify as resilience habits. My contribution to the conversation is to view all of these things through the lens of redox systems and their role in stress resilience and adaptation, hence the phrase 'redox self-care.' I hope you will find the perspective useful, but feel free to supplement this material with others' wisdom and experience. I won't be offended.

Defining Your Resilience Habits

While I'm awed by the progress science is making in understanding the body and its systems, I'm also struck by the wisdom of ancient cultures and how many resilience practices have long histories in world religions and diverse cultures. A short list would include **fasting** (all major religions), **intermittent fasting** (Islam/Ramadan, Lent), **vegetarianism** (Hinduism, Buddhism, Jainism, Seventh Day Adventists), **prayer/meditation** (all major religions), **yoga** has its roots in India, c. 2700 BCE, **quigong** and **tai chi** have long histories in China, **heat/cold stress** from Nordic countries where 10-20 minutes in the sauna is customarily followed by a run or swim in the cold. **Tea drinking** from India, China, and Japan, **coffee drinking** from Ethiopia, **yerba maté** drinking from Paraguay, **dancing,** and **fermented foods** from nearly all cultures. As you choose your resilience habits, enjoy the richness of options and variety world cultures have contributed.

A useful collection of resilience habits begins with a strong foundation of three core resilience practices, starting with sleep.

Core Resilience Habit #1: Sleep

Sleep is an evolutionarily conserved activity. Most animals do it, despite the risk from predators and the obvious reality that you aren't foraging or procreating when you're sleeping. That's a strong indication of its importance. Sleep plays critical roles in learning, memory, emotional regulation, attention, creativity, decision-making, immune function, inflammation, autonomic function (e.g., heart rate, breathing, blood pressure, body temperature), hormonal regulation (e.g., leptin, ghrelin, insulin, cortisol). According to the National Sleep foundation, human adults need 7-9 hours of quality sleep, babies and children need more for developmental reasons, and adults over 65 should get 7-8 hours. When we don't sleep enough or our sleep is disturbed or dysregulated, we're vulnerable to a wide variety of health issues and disease, including metabolic syndrome, diabetes, heart disease, arrhythmias, heart attack, stroke, obesity, hypertension, anxiety, depression, asthma, COPD, cancer, and death.[110]

While it's fair to say that sleep is still not fully understood, the "free radical flux theory of sleep" posits that sleep is, in essence, an antioxidant for the brain.[111] Oxidants accumulate during waking hours and are detoxified during sleep. The connection between dysregulated sleep and oxidative stress is clear and supported by a growing body of research. High-quality sleep of sufficient duration is a de-stressor, providing both time and mechanisms for cellular repair, waste clearance, rebalancing of the autonomic nervous system, immune system, endocrine system, and redox systems.

Sleep deprivation and dysregulation cause increased oxidative stress levels, though the underlying mechanisms can vary based on what is disturbing your sleep. Repeated hypoxic events from sleep apnea upregulate hypoxia-inducible factor 1a (HIF1a), which upregulates NADPH-oxidase (NOX4) with a resulting increase in ROS production and oxidative stress. Research into noise from aircraft during sleep showed it disrupted circadian rhythms, which downregulated FOXO3 (a major longevity gene), leading to increased oxidative stress and inflammation via upregulated NOX2 and eNOS.

---

110 Bonsignore, M.R., Baiamonte, P., Mazzuca, E. *et al.* "Obstructive sleep apnea and comorbidities: a dangerous liaison." *Multidiscip Respir Med* 14, 8 (2019). doi:10.1186/s40248-019-0172-9

111 Reimund, E. "The free radical flux theory of sleep." *Medical hypotheses* vol. 43,4 (1994): 231-3. doi:10.1016/0306-9877(94)90071-x

In addition to sound and breathing disruption, sleep can be disrupted by many other stimuli and conditions, including
- Tobacco use
- Caffeine
- Medications (e.g., hypertension meds, SSRI antidepressants, antihistamines)
- Blue light spectrum from screens
- Sympathetic hyperactivation
- Psychosocial stress
- Enlarged prostate/frequent urination
- Eating or drinking before bed
- Strenuous exercise before bed
- Chronic pain
- Neuropathy
- Anxiety
- Depression

Sleep experts promote the idea of "sleep hygiene," healthy sleep habits that promote your ability to fall asleep and stay asleep. Typical recommendations for useful sleep hygiene practices include
- Establish a sleep routine that includes going to bed and rising at close to the same time daily, even on vacations and weekends. Pre-bedtime rituals can also be useful (e.g., warm shower, prayer/meditation).
- Avoid exposure to screens before bedtime, as blue light emissions can disrupt circadian rhythms that govern sleep.
- Avoid naps if possible, particularly if you are having difficulty falling asleep at night.
- Create a mental expectation that bed is for sleeping and sex. Don't read, watch TV or play games in bed. If you can't get to sleep in 20 minutes, get up. Go to bed when you are sleepy.
- Keep the bedroom pleasant, dark, and cool. Eliminate LEDs and other light sources if possible. If your partner snores address the issue.
- Reduce fluid intake before bedtime.

- Avoid substances or activities that might interfere with sleep (e.g., tobacco, alcohol, caffeine, large meals, prescription meds).

Despite increasing knowledge about sleep and sleep pathologies, insomnia and sleep disorders have become a global problem, affecting up to 43% of the world's population by some estimates.[112] Those most vulnerable include
- Women. Up to 67% of women reported multiple nights of poor sleep in the past month. Insomnia rates for women are twice that of men.
- Older adults with short sleep and long sleep increasing the risk of mortality.
- Shift workers, those whose work involves frequent time zone changes, and students with irregular sleep schedules. These groups are vulnerable to disruptions of the circadian clock.
- Those with underlying issues including chronic illness, sleep apnea, and restless leg syndrome.

Just as disrupted or insufficient sleep can cause poor mental and physical health, underlying health issues can manifest themselves as sleep-related symptoms such as daytime sleepiness, inattention, and loss of focus, problems going to sleep, short or long sleep, sleep fragmentation, excessive napping. Indeed, sleep issues and oxidative stress can become a proinflammatory feedforward loop. Stress/oxidative stress causes disordered sleep, disordered sleep causes further oxidative stress, and so forth, leading to increased disease symptom frequency and severity. On the plus side, our collection of stress resilience habits should promote healthy sleep, creating a virtual circle.

---

112 Chattu, Vijay Kumar et al. "The Global Problem of Insufficient Sleep and Its Serious Public Health Implications." *Healthcare (Basel, Switzerland)* vol. 7,1 1. 20 Dec. 2018, doi:10.3390/healthcare7010001

Sleep Interventions

Because of the importance of sleep to overall mental and physical health, if you recognize that you are having sleep problems, you'll want to address them, either through improved sleep hygiene (see above) or through some of these additional strategies:

- **Addressing low vitamin D status.** A 2018 meta-analysis of prior research showed that people with low vitamin D status (< 20 ng/mL) had a 1.5x increased risk of sleep disorders than the high vitamin D status group.[113] Furthermore, intervention studies have shown improvements to sleep quality and duration when these deficits are addressed through supplementation. For those with restless leg syndrome, addressing low vitamin D status may improve RLS symptoms as well.[114]
- **Addressing low magnesium status.** In addition to its role as a glutathione cofactor, magnesium assists in converting vitamin D to its active (1,25[OH]2D) form and upregulates GABA, giving it a potential role in sleep issues. While studies show varied results, in an 8-week study of elderly patients, magnesium supplementation (500 mg/daily) improved subjective and objective measures of insomnia.[115]
- **Regular aerobic exercise and strength training.** In population studies, those with fitness routines, including strength and aerobic training, reported fewer sleep-related problems.

---

113 Gao, Qi et al. "The Association between Vitamin D Deficiency and Sleep Disorders: A Systematic Review and Meta-Analysis." *Nutrients* vol. 10,10 1395. 1 Oct. 2018, doi:10.3390/nu10101395

114 Wali, Siraj et al. "The Association Between Vitamin D Level and Restless Legs Syndrome: A Population-aBased Case-Control Study." *Journal of clinical sleep medicine : JCSM : official publication of the American Academy of Sleep Medicine* vol. 14,4 557-564. 15 Apr. 2018, doi:10.5664/jcsm.7044

115 Abbasi, Behnood et al. "The effect of magnesium supplementation on primary insomnia in elderly: A double-blind placebo-controlled clinical trial." *Journal of research in medical sciences : the official journal of Isfahan University of Medical Sciences* vol. 17,12 (2012): 1161-9.

- **Glycine supplementation.** Taking 3 grams of the amino acid glycine before bedtime has been shown to improve sleep quality and duration, reducing daytime sleepiness and fatigue.[116]
- **Melatonin supplementation.** Melatonin is a naturally occurring hormone produced by the pineal gland and in the digestive tract that is involved in regulating the circadian clock and sleep-wake cycles. Melatonin levels fall with age; thus, in Europe, it's an approved therapy for primary insomnia for adults over 55. However, clinical studies have shown efficacy treating sleep disorders in other populations, including children with ADHD, children with autism, teens with depression, adults with hypertension taking beta-blockers, etc.). Because melatonin is a potent antioxidant with system-wide effects, it has benefits beyond regulation of sleep, reducing risks of heart disease, diabetes, kidney disease, and other diseases associated with sleep disorders.[117] Melatonin is safe and well-tolerated, particularly compared to commercial sleep aids. Typical dosing recommendations start with a low dose, 0.5 - 1 mg two hours before bed, and raise as needed in 1-2 mg increments.
- **GABA/L-theanine supplementation.** A 2018 mouse study showed that the combination of GABA (γ-Aminobutyric acid) and l-theanine, an amino acid found in tea, worked synergistically to improve sleep quality and duration.[118] A small 2020 human study with autistic children, who as a group experience high rates of sleep

---

116 Bannai, Makoto et al. "The effects of glycine on subjective daytime performance in partially sleep-restricted healthy volunteers." *Frontiers in neurology* vol. 3 61. 18 Apr. 2012, doi:10.3389/fneur.2012.00061

117 Zizhen Xie, Fei Chen, William A. Li, Xiaokun Geng, Changhong Li, Xiaomei Meng, Yan Feng, Wei Liu & Fengchun Yu. "A review of sleep disorders and melatonin." *Neurological Research*. 39:6, 559-565, 2017. doi: 10.1080/01616412.2017.1315864

118 Kim, Suhyeon et al. "GABA and l-theanine mixture decreases sleep latency and improves NREM sleep." *Pharmaceutical biology* vol. 57,1 (2019): 65-73. doi:10.1080/13880209.2018.1557698

disorders, showed that administering GABA with Oolong tea improved anxiety, balance, and sensorimotor skills.[119] The above interventions suggest that along with good sleep hygiene and resilience practices, addressing common nutritional deficits or imbalances can improve sleep quality and minimize the oxidative stress-driven pathologies associated with disordered sleep.

Core Resilience Habit #2: Regular Exercise

In 2020, the World Health Organization (WHO) updated its physical activity guidelines for the first time in a decade.[120] What caught people's attention was what changed from the 2010 guidelines, which included:
- Elimination of minimum durations. The 2010 guidelines had specified a minimum period of 10 minutes. The message? All movement is important!
- Increased emphasis on reducing sedentary time. Some of this was population-focused: pregnant and postpartum women, the disabled, and those with chronic conditions like diabetes and hypertension. Children and teens are advised to limit screen time. But generally, being sedentary is a problem, and no one gets a pass.
- Adults are strongly encouraged to get 150-300 minutes of moderate exercise or 75-150 minutes of vigorous aerobic exercise weekly. For children, the recommendation is 60 minutes of moderate to vigorous activity daily.
- Older adults are advised to get a mix of moderate or greater strength and balance training three or more days per week to prevent falls and maintain function.

---

119 Hannant, Penelope et al. "A double-blind, placebo-controlled, randomised-designed GABA tea study in children diagnosed with autism spectrum conditions: a feasibility study clinical trial registration: ISRCTN 72571312." *Nutritional neuroscience* vol. 24,1 (2021): 45-61. doi:10.1080/1028415X.2019.1588486

120 Bull FC, Al-Ansari SS, Biddle S, et al. "World Health Organization 2020 guidelines on physical activity and sedentary behaviour." *British Journal of Sports Medicine* 2020;54:1451-1462.

- Strength training gets increased emphasis.

While the role of oxidative stress and redox signaling in exercise adaptation hasn't hit the WHO radar, these guidelines largely align with what I'm about to present.

The Perils of Inactivity

The body needs to move. In college, I helped a quadriplegic floormate with his daily physical therapy, which included stretching out leg muscles that would otherwise draw up entirely, making simple tasks like dressing and sitting in his chair difficult or impossible. It was a striking introduction to the health hazards of inactivity, forced or voluntary. To further illustrate this, the list of pathologies growing out of bed-rest is long and includes[121]

- Muscle loss/weakness
- Bone loss/weakness
- Bedsores
- Blood clots
- Increased resting heart rate
- Postural hypotension (low blood pressure upon standing/changing position)
- Shortening of muscles, tendons, and ligaments
- Joint inflexibility
- Increased pneumonia risk
- Increased risk of urinary tract infections
- Loss of appetite
- Reduced sense of taste and smell
- Constipation

Recent attention to the risks of sitting (sitting is the new smoking!) grew out of similar observations that prolonged sitting carried health risks similar to obesity and smoking that were not entirely offset by regular exercise. This notion has reached my Apple watch, which now prods me to stand hourly for at least a minute—enshrined as one of the three 'rings'

---

121 Kehler, D S et al. "Bed rest and accelerated aging in relation to the musculoskeletal and cardiovascular systems and frailty biomarkers: A review." *Experimental gerontology* vol. 124 (2019): 110643. doi:10.1016/j.exger.2019.110643

alongside exercise and movement. Does that approach work? There's some evidence to support it, including a clinical study that showed people who replaced sitting with two minutes of light exercise per hour had a 33% reduction in mortality throughout the study.[122] Closer to home, my father's blood clots, which ultimately caused his death at age 85, were very likely caused by his penchant for watching US Open Tennis hour after hour on cable TV.

What We Are Learning About Exercise

This long list of pathologies illustrates how our bodies depend on the regular hormetic and de-stressing effects of movement to maintain healthy function across all bodily systems. But how best to leverage exercise as an oxidative eustressor/resilience habit is subject to much debate in large part because every person's goals, life situation, needs, and body, are different. We are awash in information about exercise, such that you could easily be excused for being confused. In the supermarket checkout, I see a never-ending stream of formulaic articles for the <insert number here> minute workout guaranteed to firm your <insert body part here> and help you <insert desirable goal here> in just <insert improbably short time interval here>. But given that the National Enquirer is probably not the best source of health information, let's start with what we generally know to be true about exercise:

Exercise is (the Best) Medicine

The idea that exercise is medicine has penetrated deeply enough into the national psyche that it gets serious discussion in both popular and medical circles. The analogy works because exercise as a therapy should be *prescribed*—a specific *modality* at specific *dosage*, *frequency*, and *formulation*—with specific goals and outcomes in mind: improved aerobic

---

122 Beddhu, Srinivasan et al. "Light-intensity physical activities and mortality in the United States general population and CKD subpopulation." *Clinical journal of the American Society of Nephrology : CJASN* vol. 10,7 (2015): 1145-53. doi:10.2215/CJN.08410814

capacity, strength, endurance, flexibility, and balance. Like medicine, high doses can be toxic and low doses ineffective. The responses to the exercise can vary greatly between individuals, thus the need to tailor the exercise to the needs of the specific person.

With the above caveats in mind, regular moderate exercise outdoes its pharmaceutical counterparts by preventing disease through a broad range of effects including
- Lowering baseline oxidative stress levels.
- Improving antioxidant capacity and resilience to future stressors.
- Lowering baseline pain status.
- Reducing DNA damage and oxidative damage in response to exercise.
- Stimulating mitochondrial biogenesis, resulting in more, healthier mitochondria, and increased energy.
- Maintaining and increasing muscle mass.
- Maintaining and increasing bone density.
- Maintaining or improving autonomic balance.
- Improving strength and endurance (exercise capacity).
- Inducing useful epigenetic modifications to DNA and histone methylation, histone acetylation, and miRNA expression positively impact diabetes, heart disease, blood pressure, respiratory diseases, cancer, and genetically driven diseases.

There are Four Classes of Exercise

Strength, endurance, balance, and flexibility are all classes of exercise—and it's important to get a mix of all four regularly—particularly as you age.

Trained Athletes (Aerobic and Anaerobic) are More Resilient to Exercise-induced Oxidative Stress than the Untrained

This is perhaps a 'well duh' statement, but proving the intuitively obvious notion that exercise improves resilience is useful. It has been measured using oxidative stress biomarkers we discussed in chapter 5.

There's No Such Thing as 'Too Old to Exercise'

Everything we think of as the hallmarks of aging—frailty, muscle loss, bone loss, cognitive decline, reduced energy, lowered immunity, loss of balance, even declines in vision and hearing—are slowed or reversed by exercise. This is true because exercise addresses the underlying cellular issues associated with these declines, including

- Genomic instability
- Telomere attrition/shortening
- Epigenetic alterations
- Loss of proteostasis
- Dysregulated nutrient sensing
- Mitochondrial dysfunction
- Cellular senescence
- Stem cell exhaustion
- Altered intercellular communication[123]

As a general principle, in exercise, these benefits accrue via redox signaling-driven activation of NRF2 and the adaptive upregulation of antioxidant defenses. This has been demonstrated in multiple studies of exercise in NRF2 knockout mice (mice genetically unable to produce NRF2). The knockout mice experienced the stress of exercise without the adaptive benefits. Since NRF2 levels fall with age, it is reasonable to assume that exercise dosing and peak exertion should lower as we age.

Interval Training is Useful

The idea that short bursts of exercise, followed by longer periods of recovery, increases exercise benefits has gained popularity and scientific backing. It also aligns well with the concepts of hormesis and eustress. Short doses of elevated physical stress efficiently and effectively induce a useful adaptive response without crossing over into distress.

---

[123] Rebelo-Marques, Alexandre et al. "Aging Hallmarks: The Benefits of Physical Exercise." *Frontiers in endocrinology* vol. 9 258. 25 May. 2018, doi:10.3389/fendo.2018.00258

Adaptations May Be Necessary, and That's Fine

Any exercise regime that qualifies as a resilience habit has some basic requirements:
1. That you do it regularly (persistence)
2. That it makes you more resilient (growth)
3. That it doesn't injure you (sustainability)

To achieve those basics, you may need to make adaptations. Using my own experience to illustrate:

- **Persistence**
  - I'm more likely to exercise if it doesn't involve driving to the gym, so I'm drawn to running or walking in my neighborhood and biking quiet streets and trails.
  - I enjoy walking and biking with my wife, but running works less well for various reasons. And for biking, the only reason it works is that we bought a tandem so that our individual differences and collective efforts are feeding a single drivetrain—an enforced togetherness that works for us. Biking also benefits from having the right equipment: padded gloves, a helmet, padded shorts, biking shoes, a hitch-mounted rack to transport the tandem.
  - I live in Indiana, which means I have to vary my fitness routine to accommodate the blazing August heat and the sub-zero cold of January/February. That requires multiple strategies, including running in the morning in the summer and shifting to the afternoon in the winter, cultivating indoor and outdoor routines, driving south when a 10-degree temperature increase makes the difference between biking and not biking.
  - Listening to audiobooks is a guilty pleasure for me, so combining it with my daily walk/run is an inducement to get out and do it.
- **Growth**
  - I'm an Apple watch user, but fitness trackers start at under $25. With the help of the watch, I'm tracking various biomarkers that are relevant to my health situation:

- **Resting heart rate** (autonomic balance, cardiovascular fitness). In the last year, I've dropped from near 90 to routinely under 70 beats per minute.
- **Heart rate variability** (autonomic balance, cardiovascular fitness). In the last year, this has risen from an average of 19 ms to 45 ms.
- **Blood pressure** (autonomic balance, cardiovascular fitness) This has gone from borderline high (140/90) to normal (120/78). I have a separate cuff to measure this.
- **Weight.** (Metabolic health) In the last six months, I've lost 25 lbs. I still have 45 lbs to go. Exercise alone won't solve this, but it helps.
- **Neutrophil/Lymphocyte Ratio/NLR** (Oxidative Stress/Inflammation/Resilience). At my last physical, my NLR was 2.0, which is serving as a baseline. My goal is to get it down to 1.6.
- **VO2 Max** (cardiovascular fitness). The Apple Watch and other fitness bands use a metric known as "Predicted VO2 Max" based on heart activity during exercise. This approach is less accurate than a treadmill test at the hospital but has the advantage of being free and frequently updated. In my experience, this value barely budges, though I've finally gotten it to move to above average for my age after sustained daily workouts. Exercise and weight loss will both help improve VO2 Max.

The business truism, "That which is measured, improves," applies to fitness, so I encourage you to take advantage of our unprecedented ability to measure an ever-expanding collection of health parameters continuously.

- **Sustainability**
  - I'm still overweight and, at age 60, have some concerns about joint damage and other injuries, so I favor low-impact exercise such as walking and cycling, and when I run, it's still not very far, yet!

- Using the formula (220 - age = maximum heart rate), I have adjusted my workouts to stay below this threshold, which for me is 160. The Apple's Fitness+ feature that displays your heart rate on the screen as you work out is very useful for monitoring this and has become my go-to for indoor exercising.
- I've never been flexible, so when I do yoga, I have to accept that I have limitations in how far I can stretch, poses I can't do, and take satisfaction in small improvements, which are indeed happening.

You can probably think of many others in your own life, but whatever adaptations make exercising possible, enjoyable, motivational, sustainable, and relevant to your health maintenance and improvement—make them! You may also have figured out from my various biomarkers that I'm working on getting out of a health status hole that took 60 years to dig! If I can motivate some people by being ordinary, that's great. While I take some solace in knowing that when my grandfather was my age, he'd been dead ten years, I still aspire to be exemplary—to apply what I'm learning to turn back the clock on aging and make my remaining years as full, fun and productive as possible, to maximize not just lifespan, but healthspan.

Dosing Matters

Everyone moves. How you move—how often, how long, how intense—will determine whether your regimen (or lack thereof) enhances or harms your health. Scientific consensus on exercise dosing is hard to come by, because at a population level there is no one correct answer. Nevertheless, several basic principles are emerging:
- Contracting muscles produce ROS.
- ROS plays a role in muscle fatigue.
- Redox signaling produces the body's adaptive response to exercise, and this occurs primarily in the post-exercise recovery period.
- Exercise dosing is biphasic—low doses are beneficial, high doses have declining benefits, and can be toxic. A recent

study of runners showed the benefits falling off at 100 minutes/day of moderate exercise
- Oxidative stress blood biomarkers peak 0-4 hours after exercise and typically return to baseline after 6 hours.[124]
- Exercise training raises superoxide dismutase 2 (SOD2) levels, which is cardioprotective.

Timing Matters

Human biology is significantly regulated by multiple clock mechanisms, the most prominent being the circadian clock located in the suprachiasmatic nucleus of the brain's hypothalamus. Indeed, multiple studies have shown a link between circadian disruption in shift workers and metabolic syndrome, diabetes, obesity, cardiovascular disease, and more recently, a 1.7x increase in sarcopenia (muscle loss).[125] While the research is still immature, the emerging picture is one where:

- Muscle tissue has its own circadian clocks, part of the larger peripheral clock of the circadian system.
- Exercise upregulates clock genes (Bmal1, Cry1, and Per2) and can at least partially re-regulate circadian rhythms disrupted by age and shift work.
- Timed exercise can induce circadian phase shifts, effectively changing when our sleep/wake cycle occurs. A shift advance means you'll need sleep earlier, while a shift delay means the cycle will begin later. How exercise affects phase shift depends on whether you are a night owl (late chronotype) or an early bird (early chronotype). In a 2019 study, late chronotypes, who typically have the greatest circadian disruption, experienced a shift advance from morning and evening exercise. Early chronotypes

---

[124] Kawamura, Takuji, and Isao Muraoka. "Exercise-Induced Oxidative Stress and the Effects of Antioxidant Intake from a Physiological Viewpoint." *Antioxidants (Basel, Switzerland)* vol. 7,9 119. 5 Sep. 2018, doi:10.3390/antiox7090119

[125] Choi, Youn I et al. "Circadian rhythm disruption is associated with an increased risk of sarcopenia: a nationwide population-based study in Korea." Scientific reports vol. 9,1 12015. 19 Aug. 2019, doi:10.1038/s41598-019-48161-w

experienced a shift advance from morning exercise but a shift delay from evening exercise.[126] This aligns with conventional warnings not to exercise too close to bedtime while affirming that exercise can be useful in reregulating our circadian clock.
- Mitochondrial function is connected to circadian rhythms, with some evidence indicating that exercise performance peaks in the late afternoon. There also seem to be benefits to exercising at a consistent time.
- Timed exercise can elicit maximal health benefits. A 2020 publication showed diabetic/pre-diabetic men exercising in the afternoon experienced superior results compared to their morning exercising counterparts. The increased benefits included improved glucose control, fasting plasma glucose levels, exercise performance, and fat mass.[127]

Resting and Recovery Matters

Exercise involves catabolic and anabolic processes—breaking down fats and carbohydrates during exercise to produce energy, building up muscle, and repairing micro-injuries post-exercise. What is broken down in exertion must be built back up in recovery. Exercise also impacts sympathetic and parasympathetic tone in the autonomic nervous system. Exercise upregulates sympathetic activity during the workout but enhances parasympathetic tone in the post-exercise recovery and resting phase. Indeed, physical fitness hallmarks—low resting heart rate, greater heart rate variability, quicker heart rate recovery post-exercise, optimal blood pressure—are all indicators of enhanced parasympathetic tone (aka vagal tone) and all improve with exercise training.

---

126 Thomas, J Matthew et al. "Circadian rhythm phase shifts caused by timed exercise vary with chronotype." JCI insight vol. 5,3 e134270. 13 Feb. 2020, doi:10.1172/jci.insight.134270

127 Mancilla, Rodrigo et al. "Exercise training elicits superior metabolic effects when performed in the afternoon compared to morning in metabolically compromised humans." *Physiological reports* vol. 8,24 (2021): e14669. doi:10.14814/phy2.14669

By highlighting anabolic/catabolic and sympathetic/parasympathetic axes in exercise, I'm drawing your attention to several important truths:

- If you are just starting your exercise habit, you are more likely to have a sympathetic/parasympathetic imbalance and lack the resilience adaptations that a trained individual has already gained. Thus, you must start slowly, with lower exertion and longer recovery periods, or risk experiencing your exercise as a stressor rather than a eustressor.
- Psychological stress or inadequate recovery can put even someone who trains regularly into a sympathetic/parasympathetic imbalance. Exercise physiologists are increasingly using heart rate variability (HRV) as a tool for measuring sympathetic/parasympathetic imbalance to assess recovery from prior workouts, diagnose overtraining and prescribe training of appropriate intensity to athletes.[128] Average consumers can leverage smartwatches, fitness trackers, Bluetooth heart monitors, and blood pressure cuffs to measure and track resting heart rate, HRV, heart rate recovery, and blood pressure. This is useful for understanding autonomic and sympathetic/parasympathetic balance, which along with improved cardiometabolic health and fitness, is a goal of exercise as a resilience habit.
- Adequate recovery is a necessary component of any exercise regimen and will vary with fitness level, exercise type, intensity, duration, redox, and autonomic status. Know your body. Listen to it. Exercising when sick, injured, or not fully recovered from over-exertion is more likely to push your exercise beyond eustress into oxidative distress.

Exercise: Wrapping Up

Everyone moves, but getting the right combination of activity type, frequency, intensity, and duration determines whether

---

128 Dong, J."The role of heart rate variability in sports physiology (Review)". Experimental and Therapeutic Medicine 11.5 (2016): 1531-1536.

that movement confers resilience or contributes to aging and chronic disease. Exercise as a eustressor is an emerging concept, where oxidative stress and redox signaling activate NRF2 and invoke an adaptive response that increases resilience to future stress. The hormetic effects of exercise are as essential to health and wellness as eating and sleeping. We increasingly understand the interrelatedness of these activities, where each plays a role in maintaining resilience, optimal metabolic function and energy production, immune, hormonal balance, and nutritional and redox status. And that brings us to resilience habit #3.

Core Resilience Habit #3: A Nutrient-dense Diet

Just as everyone moves, all humans eat. Yet we are confronted with undeniable evidence that wherever in the world the western diet goes, the diseases of western civilization follow. A lot of ink has been spilled on this topic, but the core sins of the western diet that make it a primary driver of redox imbalance and downstream chronic disease include

- Overconsumption of low-nutrient processed carbs and sugars
- Overconsumption of meat—beef and cured meats in particular
- Overconsumption of grain oils with a resulting omega 3-6 imbalance.
- Overconsumption of dairy products[129]
- Overconsumption of food additives and preservatives
- Underconsumption of fruits, vegetables, leafy greens, nuts, seeds, legumes
- Underconsumption of prebiotic fiber and resistant starch.
- Underconsumption of fermented foods.

The impact of these dietary sins are many:
- Hyperinsulinemia

---

129 The role of dairy in diet is controversial. While earlier health concerns were focused on saturated fat, more recent attention has been given to possible health impacts of D-galactose, casein and IGF-1, as well as the role of milk proteins as allergens. For people seeking anti-inflammatory diets, I generally advise avoiding dairy, at least initially.

- Insulin resistance
- Redox imbalance
- Inflammation
- Metabolic damage
- Obesity
- A pro-inflammatory microbiome
- Increased intestinal permeability
- Increased vascular permeability
- Chronic immune system activation
- Immune system dysregulation/autoimmunity
- Lowered nutritional status

All of the above lead to the chronic diseases of aging and reduced lifespan/health span.

Making Your Diet a Resilience Habit

Diets can easily be stressors. Thus, making your diet a resilience habit involves reducing or eliminating the dietary stressors listed above and incorporating the nutrient-dense foods and dietary eustressors that bolster nutritional status and confer resilience. Unsurprisingly, most of the eustressors and nutrient-dense foods are plants. Research into why plant-based diets prevent disease has identified thousands of phytonutrients that function as low-level stressors that upregulate resilience pathways, including NRF2, AMPK, PGC1a and FOXO. It's worth pointing out that exercise also upregulates NRF2, AMPK, PGC1a, and FOXO pathways, invoking epigenetic changes to several hundred genes related to cellular defense and stress resilience.

While studies have isolated an increasing number of highly useful polyphenols, terpenoids, alkaloids, phytosterols, and organosulfur compounds that can be used as nutritional supplements, eating whole foods has the benefit of delivering a much broader array of phytonutrients that may act synergistically even at lower concentrations. While this is difficult to prove through reductionist approaches, observational studies of plant-based diets largely bear this out.

Why Focus on Nutrient Density?

While nutrient-dense diets are largely plant-based, the notion of nutrient density has many advantages. First, it provides a basis for avoiding the 'junk-food vegan' trap, where the food industry plies you with low-nutrient, processed foods labeled as vegan-friendly. Second and more importantly, stress in all its forms incurs a nutritional cost that can affect nutritional status and redox and immune status. Eating nutrient-dense foods helps replenish lost nutrients and maintain healthy redox and immune status. Knowing that you are experiencing elevated stress levels can also allow you to develop nutritional intervention strategies to mitigate those stressors. Third, focusing on nutrient density avoids debates over macronutrient ratios (proteins, fats, carbohydrates) Finally, the labels we put on our dietary strategies have a near-religious dimension which isn't always helpful. Nutrient-density is a less doctrinaire label, leaving open the use of animal foods if it makes sense to do so. Eating fish periodically, in particular, seems to have useful nutritional benefits that go beyond what an entirely plant-based diet can offer. Ultimately, paying attention to nutrient density can improve the quality of most any dietary -ism you might choose.

But what about <insert hot new diet here>?

The health section of your bookstore is populated with LOTS of books on diet—more than I can address or critique, but several are worth touching on.

Paleo Diets

I know many people who have done well on paleo diets, particularly those with autoimmune/allergy issues. Paleo diets purport to eliminate foods our paleolithic ancestors wouldn't have eaten and thus are whole food, minimally processed diets. This has the important benefit of eliminating processed carbs, refined sugars, food additives, and grain oils from your diet—the elements driving the bulk of inflammation in the western diet. Grains and beans/legumes are off-limits, which can be useful for anyone with gluten sensitivity or lectin intolerance. And dairy products are off-limits, which removes yet another common allergen. A 2019 review of the impact of diet types on the microbiome showed paleo diets improving microbial diversity, which is important for gut barrier health and inflammatory status.[130]

Potential concerns about the paleo diet are primarily focused on sustainability, getting adequate fiber and resistant starch when beans and grains are off-limits, and whether trading meat for beans as a primary protein source is a good health deal in the long term. High meat consumption is linked with cancer,[131] and beans are an important source of soluble fiber, promoting the production of health-inducing short-chain fatty acids in the gut. That said, I do believe that paleo diets can be consonant with the goal of making your diet a resilience practice.

Ketogenic Diets

Ketogenic diets (KDs) focus on high fat consumption to put your body into ketosis, where the body burns fat for fuel. The classic keto diet prescribes a 3-4:1 ratio of fat to protein+carbs. Research has shown ketogenic diets to produce short term oxidative stress that activates NRF2 and an adaptive response that can be beneficial particularly in brain function and memory. This makes ketogenic diets a potential resilience practice, but one that is largely incompatible with plant-centric diets, which have a much stronger track record for disease prevention and reversal. Nevertheless, emerging evidence on ketogenic diets shows benefits in weight loss, metabolic function, insulin sensitivity, and neuroinflammatory

---

130 Klement, Rainer J, and Valerio Pazienza. "Impact of Different Types of Diet on Gut Microbiota Profiles and Cancer Prevention and Treatment." *Medicina (Kaunas, Lithuania)* vol. 55,4 84. 29 Mar. 2019, doi:10.3390/medicina55040084

131 Pelland-St-Pierre, Laura et al. "Genotoxic effect of meat consumption: A mini review." *Mutation research* vol. 863-864 (2021): 503311. doi:10.1016/j.mrgentox.2021.503311

conditions. These benefits are mediated by KDs ability to invoke a hormetic/eustress response.[132]

Recent evidence has highlighted intermittent fasting's ability to induce ketosis, specifically time-restricted feeding, where eating occurs in an abbreviated time window. This may be an attractive alternative to full-blown ketogenic diets, which necessarily miss out on some of the hormetic benefits of plant-based eating. We'll explore this more later in the chapter.

Diet Wrap-up

What you eat or don't eat and how much largely determines the extent to which your diet is a resilience practice. Author Michael Pollan's aphorism "Eat [real] food, not too much, mostly plants," comes close to capturing the goal of diet as a resilience practice. That this is so difficult to achieve goes beyond any one individual's poor choices or lack of willpower.

The problem includes Ag policy and school lunch programs that prioritize cheap food over nutritious food, federal nutrition guidelines that are beholden to the meat and dairy lobby, a medical education curriculum that is light on nutrition, a healthcare system that still undervalues lifestyle interventions, a food industry that sells us products that are cheap, convenient, tasty and have a long shelf life but ultimately undermine our health, restaurant portions that are 'all-you-can-eat' or twice what you should be eating. Eating for resilience in this environment can be done but requires commitment, intentionality, and at times the wholesale retraining of our taste buds and eating habits.

I put diet in the number three position of the core resilience habits for a reason. Many health books treat diet as though it was the only thing that mattered, and that simply isn't true. Our three-legged resilience stool depends on sleep, diet, and exercise, and each is essential to future health and stress

---

132 Pinto A, Bonucci A, Maggi E, Corsi M, Businaro R. "Anti-Oxidant and Anti-Inflammatory Activity of Ketogenic Diet: New Perspectives for Neuroprotection in Alzheimer's Disease." *Antioxidants*. 2018; 7(5):63. https://doi.org/10.3390/antiox7050063

resilience. With that solid foundation, we can now move on to address lesser-known resilience habits that build on that foundation to keep illness, aging, and chronic disease at bay.

Resilience Habit: Stay Hydrated

Humans are generally over 50% water, and staying hydrated is most certainly an under-appreciated health practice. Studies have shown dehydration in the elderly raises healthcare costs, increases mortality and frailty, reduces cognitive function, impacts oral and joint health, and increases the risk of transient ischemic attacks (TIAs) and strokes.[133] At any age, staying hydrated is important for joint, muscle, and overall physical and mental health. With the superabundance of beverage choices, it bears repeating that the best choice for hydration is still water. Drinking water before meals can reduce appetite and aid in weight loss.

Research on athletes has shown that dehydration raises oxidative stress parameters, and subsequent rehydration lowers them. While water intake needs vary by gender, climate, altitude, and exertion level, most recommendations fall between 2 and 4 liters per day, which would amount to between 8 and 16 eight-ounce glasses of water daily. One study found that the body makes neuroendocrine adaptations to preserve water levels below 1.8L/day and that many people do not reach that level.

While much of the literature has quite reasonably focused on dehydration as a source of distress and subsequent damage and dysregulation, there is evidence from animal studies that acute dehydration may invoke adaptive responses in ways similar to other resilience habits via NRF2 and FOXO activation. To my knowledge, there are no human studies explicitly on dehydration and hormesis, though it's not

---

[133] Edmonds, Caroline J et al. "Dehydration in older people: A systematic review of the effects of dehydration on health outcomes, healthcare costs and cognitive performance." *Archives of gerontology and geriatrics*, vol. 95 104380. 17 Feb. 2021, doi:10.1016/j.archger.2021.104380

unreasonable to assume that there's a component of this effect occurring in exercise. At this point, the conservative advice would be to get any dehydration eustress benefits through exercise, accompanied by adequate rehydration as needed during and post-exercise.

Resilience Habit: Calorie Restriction

In 1935, scientists at Cornell University discovered that mice fed a calorie-restricted diet lived 33% longer than their well-fed counterparts. Furthermore, the calorie-restricted mice stayed youthful longer and experienced fewer age-related diseases late in life. Since then, anti-aging research into everything from bacteria to fruit flies, nematodes, and rodents has shown similar lifespan and healthspan effects. Evolutionarily, organisms are designed to procreate or survive until they can procreate. Calorie restriction in this context appears to signal that times are tough and biological resources and priorities should shift towards life extension. Recent evidence suggests that the mechanisms for calorie restriction's epigenetic benefits include our good friends NRF2, AMPK, PGC1a, and FOXO, which invoke anti-aging changes to DNA methylation, histone modifications, changes in miRNA expression, much as we saw in exercise.[134]

Evidence from history (e.g., World War 1 Denmark) and early human trials indicate that calorie restriction without malnutrition in people confers life extension and health benefits analogous to those seen in animals.[135]

Also of interest are what researchers refer to as **calorie restriction mimetics**— substances that mimic the beneficial effects of calorie restriction without the privation. The most prominent of these is resveratrol, the red wine polyphenol.

---

134 Martín-Montalvo, A et al. "NRF2, cancer and calorie restriction." *Oncogene* vol. 30,5 (2011): 505-20. doi:10.1038/onc.2010.492

135 Most, Jasper et al. "Calorie restriction in humans: An update." *Ageing research reviews* vol. 39 (2017): 36-45. doi:10.1016/j.arr.2016.08.005

There is a growing list of these compounds. It includes polyphenols and other plant compounds such as quercetin, EGCG, berberine, gallic acid, fisetin, hydroxycitric acid, curcumin, the vitamin B3 precursor nicotinamide riboside, and the drug metformin.

Resilience Habit: Intermittent Fasting

Related to calorie restriction but worthy of its own category, intermittent fasting is gaining traction as an effective strategy for not only weight loss, but preventing or ameliorating diabetes, heart disease, neurological ailments and even cancer. A recent review article studying intermittent fasting (IF) in stroke reached this eye-popping conclusion:

> "Overall, we conclude that IF promotes an adaptive (stress) response in the body that includes prevention of inflammation, better handling of oxidative stress, formation of more mitochondria, transcriptional switch to turn off neurotoxic and to turn on neuroprotective genes, as well as increase brain plasticity through neurogenesis/angiogenesis. IF was shown to protect mature neurons, and to promote regeneration and plasticity by inducing neurogenesis. Most of the studies to date indicated a beneficial effect of IF in various species. An attractive feature for adoption of IF in humans is the flexibility, as the regimen can be followed for 14 to 16 hours/day or fasting on alternate days or even normal feeding on 5 days and reduced calories on 2 days of the week. All of these adaptations are known to be beneficial by reducing the incidence and negative effects of major metabolic disorders like diabetes and hypertension, as well as subsequent diseases like heart attack, stroke, or neurodegenerative diseases."[136]

I found this study to be particularly exciting because it concretely demonstrated the resilience-enhancing effects of intermittent fasting. In mice with induced ischemia (cutting off blood flow), the damage was less, and the recovery quicker in the fasting mice compared to the controls.

---

[136] Raghu Vemuganti, Thiruma V. Arumugam. "Molecular mechanisms of intermittent fasting-induced ischemic tolerance." Conditioning Medicine 2020. 3(1): 9-17.

Like other resilience practices, intermittent fasting confers resilience via activation of NRF2, AMPK, PGC1-a, and FOXO pathways, but also in time-restricted feeding, enhances circadian regulation of the gut microbiome and downregulates the mTOR pathway, which is useful in many disease states, including diabetes, obesity, autoimmunity, cancer, and neurodegeneration. Research into time-restricted feeding highlighted that their frequent grazing contributed to continuous mTOR activation in mice with unrestricted eating.

Obesity is a growing health concern globally, and the conventional wisdom is that it is an intractable problem. There's plenty of evidence that short-term weight loss is followed by rebound weight gain. Some of the most encouraging obesity research has come in time-restricted feeding, where eating is restricted to an abbreviated time window—typically 6 to 8 hours. The shortened time window for eating has many advantages: some of the hormetic benefits of ketogenic diets without the high-fat consumption, a longer duration for rest and repair of the digestive tract, longer periods of decreased insulin release leading to reduced hyperinsulinemia, increased insulin sensitivity, and improvement in circadian clock regulation. In an obese, post-menopausal mouse study, these changes resulted in a striking inhibition of breast cancer tumor initiation, tumor progression, and metastasis.[137]

Compliance is another significant advantage of time-restricted feeding, with a recent study using an 8-9 hour eating window showing compliance on 75% of days and significant weight loss, reduced BMI, and waist circumference.[138] I see genuine excitement among researchers at the prospect of a non-pharmaceutical intervention for weight loss and metabolic health that works, is easily understood, and sustainable for patients. It's also worth noting that there's some evidence to

---

137 Das, Manasi et al. "Time-restricted feeding normalizes hyperinsulinemia to inhibit breast cancer in obese postmenopausal mouse models." *Nature communications* vol. 12,1 565. 25 Jan. 2021, doi:10.1038/s41467-020-20743-7

138 Kesztyüs, Dorothea et al. "Adherence to Time-Restricted Feeding and Impact on Abdominal Obesity in Primary Care Patients: Results of a Pilot Study in a Pre-Post Design." *Nutrients* vol. 11,12 2854. 21 Nov. 2019, doi:10.3390/nu11122854

indicate that placing the time window earlier in the day is more effective than late in the day. In a study of timed-restricted feeding in pre-diabetic men, the early feeding group (9 a.m. - 3 pm) had the best outcomes; mid-day feeding participants experienced some benefit while putting the window after 4 pm (late feeding) actually resulted in worse outcomes than controls.[139] While these are small studies, they suggest that humans are metabolically wired for early day feeding. They also support accumulating evidence that humans are clock-driven organisms that benefit from activities that reinforce rather than disrupt our circadian rhythms.

Resilience Habit: Mindfulness/Vagus Nerve Stimulation

If there's one practice associated with stress management in the popular consciousness, it would have to be mindfulness and related activities, such as prayer, meditation, and deep breathing exercises. Beyond their spiritual and psychological benefits, these activities have the physiological effect of balancing the autonomic nervous system, with benefits for heart rate, heart rate variability, breathing, blood pressure, sexual function, mood, thermal regulation, digestion, metabolism, immune function, exercise performance, and recovery—all functions related to vagal/parasympathetic tone. All of these activities fall into the category of vagus nerve stimulators. The vagus nerve connects the brain with the gut and runs through the heart, lungs, spleen, liver, and kidneys. Decreases in vagus nerve activity, known as vagal withdrawal, are associated with poor physical fitness and physiological and psychological stress and, along with sympathetic hyperactivation, are a component of autonomic imbalance (aka sympathovagal imbalance).

---

[139] Sutton, Elizabeth F et al. "Early Time-Restricted Feeding Improves Insulin Sensitivity, Blood Pressure, and Oxidative Stress Even without Weight Loss in Men with Prediabetes." *Cell metabolism* vol. 27,6 (2018): 1212-1221.e3. doi:10.1016/j.cmet.2018.04.010

If sympathovagal imbalance were considered a disease, it would be right up there with redox imbalance, affecting billions of people worldwide. Hypertension, which accounts for 500 million prescriptions and an estimated $131 billion in healthcare spending annually in the US alone,[140] can in many cases be viewed as a symptom of sympathovagal imbalance. The idea that vagus nerve stimulating activities can ameliorate this imbalance and that most of them are free, fulfilling, and even fun (e.g., laughter, singing) speaks to the value of curating a collection of vagus nerve stimulating resilience activities. A partial list includes

- **Yoga.** While it also fits well under exercise for balance, strength, and flexibility, yoga also stimulates the vagus nerve thanks to its emphasis on breathing and meditation.
- **Qigong.** While less widely known in the west than yoga, qigong is possibly the best exercise system for maintaining sympathovagal balance. You can find numerous qigong videos on YouTube, and some are explicitly focused on hypertension and circulation.
- **Deep breathing.** Lengthening your exhale is known to activate your parasympathetic system. Several breathing techniques available leverage this to improve sympathovagal balance over time, including 4:8:8 and 4:7:8 breathing and 4:8 breathing. In 4:x:8 breathing, you inhale for 4 seconds, hold your breath for 7 or 8 seconds and exhale for 8 seconds. It's important to note that rapid breathing induces hyperventilation, causing hypoxia and sympathetic activation. Similarly, 2:1 breathing (faster exhales) also activates the sympathetic nervous system. Note that some descriptions of 2:1 breathing are describing longer exhales, which stimulates parasympathetic activity.
- **Acupressure.** Leveraging the same meridians and acupoints as acupuncture, acupressure is a traditional

---

140 Kirkland, Elizabeth B et al. "Trends in Healthcare Expenditures Among US Adults With Hypertension: National Estimates, 2003-2014." *Journal of the American Heart Association* vol. 7,11 e008731. 30 May. 2018, doi:10.1161/JAHA.118.008731

Chinese medicine therapy that, with a little practice, you can do on your own to lower heart rate, blood pressure, reduce fatigue or anxiety, and relieve pain. I have used the HT-7 acupressure point (AP), located on the inner wrist on the pinky side of the hand, and the P-6 AP on the inner arm, three finger widths below the hand to lower heart rate, and they work surprisingly well.

This is only a partial list of vagus nerve stimulators. It's important to note that exercise, in general, stimulates the vagus nerve, which in part explains the improvements to vagal/parasympathetic tone in exercise training. And I would be remiss if I didn't draw attention to the role of oxidative stress in sympathetic activation and autonomic dysregulation, as well as the role of NRF2 in mediating the resilience benefits of vagus nerve stimulation.

Resilience Habit: Acute Heat Stress

The sauna came to us from Finland, where they've been in use for millennia, but acute heat exposure is common in many cultures with purported health benefits. Accumulating evidence supports this traditional view. A review article exploring the use of saunas for individuals in high-stress occupations noted a 50% reduction in heart attacks with 4-7 sauna sessions per week and a significant reduction in sudden cardiac death and blood pressure.[141] Sauna use reduced heart attacks, oxidative stress, Alzheimer's incidence, inflammation, blood pressure and providing longevity and metabolic benefits. Regular sauna use improves vagal tone and reduces sympathetic nervous system activation. At a cellular level, it activates the adaptive stress response, upregulating protective

---

141 Henderson, Kaemmer N et al. "The Cardiometabolic Health Benefits of Sauna Exposure in Individuals with High-Stress Occupations. A Mechanistic Review." *International journal of environmental research and public health* vol. 18,3 1105. 27 Jan. 2021, doi:10.3390/ijerph18031105

heat shock proteins and activating resilience pathways NRF2, PGC1a, AMPK, and FOXO, analogous to what we observed in exercise, calorie restriction and plant-based eating.

Resilience Habit: Acute Cold Stress

In Scandinavian countries, the sauna experience can be accompanied by a roll in the snow or cold water swimming, followed by more time in the sauna. Globally, interest in cold tolerance has been piqued by dutchman Wim Hof, dubbed "The Iceman," who became something of an Internet sensation by sitting in an ice bath for one hour, 52 minutes, and 42 seconds, a world record. Wim Hof demonstrated not only that cold tolerance could be developed and enhanced over time, but he also allowed researchers to monitor his vital statistics and bodily biomarkers while doing these feats, providing useful data on how he could accomplish what many assumed should be a fatal dose of cold stress. Interest in the Wim Hof method has also drawn attention to the health benefits of more modest feats, such as flipping the shower handle to COLD at the end of a hot shower.

Resilience Habit: Controlled Hypoxia

While the cold exposure in the Wim Hof method has drawn the most attention, equally significant is the breathing method, borrowed from Tibetan Tummo meditation, Tummo meaning "inner fire." The breathing method involves 30 deep breaths in about a minute, followed by holding your breath. This process is repeated three times and induces mild hypoxia through low-level hyperventilation. This mild hypoxia has hormetic effects and done over time, the breathing method improves your ability to hold your breath and contributes to improved cold tolerance. Trained Wim Hof practitioners have shown fewer inflammatory immune reactions than controls in response to a lipopolysaccharide challenge. My own admittedly limited experience with the Wim Hof method was that while I enjoyed both the breathing and the cold shower experience, it potently activated my sympathetic nervous system at a time when I was trying to reduce sympathetic activation, so I had to stop. I suspect that I could have success if I initially reduce the sessions to once or twice a week. If you try Wim Hof Method, I recommend monitoring your resting heart rate and heart rate variability to see how they are affected. Wim Hof Method and acute cold exposure certainly appear to provoke a useful adaptive response with resilience benefits if dosing is appropriate.

Resilience Habit: Regular Blood Donation

In addition to being an altruistic act that saves others' lives, donating blood is increasingly being recognized as beneficial to the donor. A 2016 paper showed increased antioxidant activity (superoxide dismutase and serum NO levels), decreased oxidative stress, and lower inflammatory markers 24 hours post-donation.[142] Regular donors are at lower risk for heart attack and certain cancers, generally have lower blood pressure, and are protected from health issues associated with excess iron.

You can donate whole blood 4 to 6 times per year, assuming adequate iron levels. However, Mayo Clinic recently changed its interval from 8 to 12 weeks as a precaution to ensure that donor ferritin levels had fully recovered. You can donate platelets every 2-4 weeks, though platelet donations' hormetic benefits are less clear.

---

142 Yunce, Muharrem, et al. "One more health benefit of blood donation: reduces acute-phase reactants, oxidants and increases antioxidant capacity." Journal of Basic and Clinical Physiology and Pharmacology, vol. 27, no. 6, 2016, pp. 653-657. doi.org/10.1515/jbcpp-2015-0111

Resilience Habit: Micro-habits

Some activities perhaps live under larger categories or don't quite merit their own habit, but are nonetheless useful habits and activities that contribute to resilience and overall health and well-being.

- **Floss!** Oral health is increasingly recognized for its role in broader health. Gingivitis and periodontal disease can be significant sources of lipopolysaccharide (aka endotoxin), which plays a key role in systemic inflammation and chronic immune system activation.
- **Oil pulling.** On the topic of oral health, oil pulling comes to us from India's Ayurvedic medical tradition. It involves swishing sesame or coconut oil around in your mouth for 15-20 minutes. It works because these oils are anti-bacterial and possess mild detergent action that helps kill bacteria where brushes can't reach. And yes, don't swallow the oil. Lipopolysaccharide from the cell walls of dead bacteria is truly toxic and pro-inflammatory.
- **Hand Hygiene.** Whatever the COVID pandemic gave us, it certainly imparted a heightened awareness of hand hygiene, from 20-second washing routines to disinfecting stations at every turn. The stakes were higher with COVID, but hand-washing has long been a foundational practice for preventing disease spread. Do it!
- **Pedicures and foot care.** We get our teeth cleaned professionally twice a year. Why not our feet? Feet, like mouths, can be problem areas for infection, thanks to issues such as athlete's foot, corns, ingrown toenails, and cracked heels. Pedicures can help catch these problems before they become serious health issues. Men, in particular, need encouragement to stay on top of foot hygiene issues, from basic nail trimming and filing to moisturizing and callus removal.
- **Tea drinking.** Every ancient culture incorporates tea from local herbs into their food culture because of their medicinal properties. Some incorporate fermentation as well. EGCG and theaflavins from green and black tea

are the most studied compounds. Still, saponins from jiaogulan tea and rosmarinic acid from mint tea are also anti-inflammatory, health-inducing compounds. Find teas you like and learn to drink them without sugar.
- **Coffee drinking.** While it's a slightly depressing statistic, coffee is the major source of polyphenols for Americans. If you drink it black and in moderation, coffee can be a resilience micro-habit. Just be aware that coffee contains on average twice as much caffeine as tea, and caffeine raises adrenaline levels and cortisol, which can exacerbate sympathovagal imbalance and interfere with sleep quality and duration.
- **Glycine.** If you really must sweeten your coffee or tea, consider glycine, a no-calorie amino acid that looks and measures like sugar. Glycine is a glutathione precursor, helps maintain muscle mass, and 3 grams taken at night has been shown to improve sleep quality.
- **Green smoothies.** A frozen banana, 8 oz of nut milk (I like coconut-almond blend), a handful of spinach, blueberries, and/or strawberries, a heaping tablespoon of cocoa, and anything else healthy you feel like adding makes a no-added-sugar-added, nutrient-dense, epicurean treat/meal replacement. The possible variants are endless.
- **Forgiveness.** The wisdom of forgiveness is that holding onto grievances has health consequences for the aggrieved while the perpetrator has often moved on. While the studies showing this were not specific to oxidative stress, the symptoms affected have well-known oxidative stress connections and are also associated with sympathetic hyperactivation. It's important to remember that forgiveness includes forgiving yourself. Any journey towards mental or physical healing will include moments of failure and self-sabotage. Learn from it, forgive yourself, and move on.
- **Social connection.** Social isolation is a stressor that can activate the HPA axis, upregulate glucocorticoids, increase oxidative stress and shorten telomeres—all hallmarks of aging. The social hormone and neuropeptide oxytocin can

prevent some of the negative impacts of social isolation. So cultivate friendships and social connection at all stages of life. They do a body good.
- **Prepare for illness and infection.** A robust, well-regulated immune system wins. It beats colds, viruses, infections and even cancer. But sometimes, your immune needs some assistance, and early intervention can help your immune system win before something more serious develops. For me, this has meant curating a collection of antimicrobial compounds and immunonutrients that have helped me beat the colds and upper respiratory infections that used to lay me low, sometimes for weeks. We'll cover this in more detail in chapter 8.
- **Prepare for aging.** Just as illness and infection are inevitable and need preparation, so is aging. So like my preparation for illness and infection, in addition to these resilience habits, I am also curating a collection of anti-aging strategies that focuses primarily on keeping glutathione and NAD+ levels up and nutritional status for key immune and redox-related nutrients optimized. Again, more on this in chapter 8.

Measuring Resilience

In chapter 6, I described neutrophil/lymphocyte ratio (NLR) as a resilience biomarker. While there is variation based on race, genetics, and other factors, measuring NLR routinely would give us our own personal resilience baseline to understand when resilience is rising or falling. While this would be useful in its own right, it's more useful still when combined with other biomarkers, including
- **Heart rate variability,** which is greater with higher fitness levels and parasympathetic activity. If it's low, raising it is a goal of your resilience habits.
- **Resting heart rate**, which should ideally be below 70. If it's not, resilience habits that target sympathovagal balance and cardiovascular fitness are good choices.

- **Blood pressure**, which should be at or below 120/80. High blood pressure responds well to plant-based diets, exercise, and vagus nerve stimulation.
- **VO2Max**, which is a measure of aerobic fitness. In aging, low VO2Max scores are associated with mortality. Below normal VO2Max scores can be targeted with aerobic exercise and weight loss.
- **Waist/height ratio (WHR)** is a more useful metric than BMI for measuring obesity, with a target of less than a 1 to 2 ratio working well for most people. A WHR greater than 1 to 2 is critiquing both your diet and your metabolism. Time-restricted feeding, nutrient-dense eating, and regular exercise help improve WHR.
- **Fasting glucose/HbA1C.** These are the gold standard biomarkers for metabolic syndrome and diabetes. If these are high for reasons other than Type 1 diabetes, they should respond to plant-based diets, exercise, and time-restricted feeding.

All of these biomarkers help you understand both the extent of your oxidative stress-driven dysregulation across multiple systems and the resilience your self-care practices are accruing. I expect our ability to track relevant biomarkers to only improve over time, with improvements to mobile technology, continuous monitoring, and lower-cost testing capabilities.

Resilience Habits: Wrapping Up

Your chosen resilience habits will form the core of your self-care strategy. You cannot do all of them. Some, like ketogenic and plant-based diets, are mutually exclusive. You may find some harder to incorporate into your current life situation than others, or perhaps just too difficult, time-consuming, or unpleasant to adopt as a habit. Nevertheless, I would encourage you to experiment with lots of them. A cold shower won't kill you, and deep breathing exercises and acupressure probably saved me a trip to the ER during one high-stress patch in my pre-retirement life.

The big takeaway here is that the combination of a robust set of resilience habits grounded in nutritional excellence, regular exercise, 6-8 hours of a high-quality sleep, and stress reduction/management protects you against disease and should move your resilience biomarkers towards numbers considered normal or even optimal for your age. Furthermore, improvement on multiple fronts is possible at any age. I believe that, at a minimum, the increasing understanding of hormetic eustressors as resilience habits points to our ability to maintain health and wellness with minimal pharmaceutical and surgical interventions well into old age.

Chapter 8

Treating Redox Imbalance

"If you ask what is the single most important key to longevity, I would have to say it is avoiding worry, stress and tension. And if you didn't ask me, I'd still have to say it."

—George Burns

Let's recap:
- Stress causes oxidative stress and redox imbalance.
- Acute low-level stressors, our resilience habits, invoke an adaptive response via redox signaling that can confer resilience to future stressors—promoting homeostasis, cardiovascular fitness, strength, faster recovery, robust immunity, lower inflammation, enhanced mental well-being, improved cognitive function, and disease-resistance.
- Chronic or excessive stress causes local and systemic redox imbalance, causing oxidative damage, pathological signaling, and nutritional imbalances leading to dysregulation of multiple systems, including the autonomic nervous system, endocrine system (e.g., HPA axis, pancreas, thyroid), renin, angiotensin, aldosterone system, immune system, gut microbiome, gut and vascular barriers, metabolism, liver, kidneys and circulatory system.
- At a cellular level, chronic redox imbalance causes DNA damage and mutations, disruptions to the cellular life

cycle, telomere shortening, senescence, and cell death. These are all hallmarks of aging.
- Chronic redox imbalance decreases resilience and leads to a chronically activated immune system, inflammation, and increased vulnerability to disease, as well as physical symptoms such as pain, rash, fatigue, loss of function and weight gain, and mental health symptoms such as anxiety, depression, impulsivity, addiction, cognitive impairment, and neurodegeneration.
- Redox balance can be restored and resilience bolstered with resulting improvements to symptoms. As systems become increasingly damaged and dysregulated, this recovery process will likely be far more complex and take longer or fail, leading to disease, disability, frailty, and death.
- Epidemiologically, redox imbalance is an "insufficient but necessary" cause in all disease, thanks to the role of redox systems and signaling in the cellular stress response and in mediating the adaptive response to cellular and systemic stress. The implication is that effectively treating redox imbalance and associated stressors will have therapeutic benefits for all disease.

This is a different way of thinking about health and disease—a different paradigm—one that I believe is profoundly empowering for patients, meaning everyone on the planet. While it should graft well onto systems like functional medicine, which already claims to be based on systems biology, or naturopathic medicine, which is holistic and prevention-oriented, your average medical doctor was not trained to think this way. That creates a dilemma for me—how should I write about treating redox imbalance when the predominant system doesn't yet recognize it as a condition to be treated?

I ultimately decided that redox imbalance represented not only a new disease, but a new disease paradigm which necessitated a new treatment paradigm. Although I am making the case that redox imbalance is a disease, I make no secret that it is currently *not* classified as a disease. If you look at the World Health Organization's International Catalog of Diseases (ICD-11), you will not find redox imbalance among the 55,000-plus listed diseases.

I'm deeply ambivalent about how important disease classification is for conditions such as redox imbalance and aging. On the one hand, disease status confers many advantages, such as treatment protocols, the search for better biomarkers and therapies, and a general gravitas that makes the medical profession take said disease seriously. On the other hand, the disease taxonomy in ICD-11 seems bloated and outmoded—designed for an earlier century when we lacked important information about how disease worked and how interconnected our bodily systems are. Rather than a network of disease and organ specialists, we need a more holistic, systems-oriented treatment paradigm that better reflects the emerging science.

A new treatment paradigm must be cognizant of and apply a broad range of new information from disciplines that didn't even exist a generation ago. Epigenetics, once scientific heresy, is now core to the understanding of gene expression and our body's ability to dynamically adapt to its environment. Epigenetic targeting of genes and their signaling pathways is still being explored for its therapeutic potential and potential risks. Foundational pathologies such as chronic activation of the sympathetic nervous system, HPA axis, immune system, and renin-angiotensin-aldosterone system, nutritional dysregulation, mitochondrial dysfunction, disrupted protein synthesis, intestinal and vascular permeability, gut dysbiosis, and redox imbalance (of course!), largely ignored or addressed only indirectly by Western clinical medicine, take center stage in the new treatment paradigm. Existing therapies are not necessarily excluded, but neither should they automatically be assumed to be in the canon of redox therapies or play the same roles as they do now.

We begin our exploration of the redox treatment paradigm with some basic concepts and the understanding that there are already new research-based, redox-friendly concepts and a body of redox therapies that are taking shape.

Concept: Comorbidities and Multimorbidities

The idea that people who have a particular disease are statistically more likely to get another related disease isn't new. The term comorbidity appeared in research publications as early as 1970. We've also alluded that people with autoimmune disease may have multimorbidities—three or more concurrent diseases.

In a redox health paradigm, the concept of comorbidities and multimorbidities is somewhat different. I've been writing about HPA axis activation, chronic immune system activation, chronic sympathetic nervous system activation, mitochondrial dysfunction, intestinal and vascular permeability, endoplasmic reticulum stress, reduced nutritional status, and it might appear as though they were happening in isolation. The reality is that multiple pathologies can occur almost simultaneously, to the point that it can be challenging to know which comes first and what causes what.

Thus, there is the potential need to address multiple issues at once. This explains why you can't just give someone N-acetylcysteine and expect them to get well because you raised their glutathione level, why pharmaceutical monotherapies (e.g., TNFα inhibitors) don't cure disease, why nutrient-dense, whole food, plant-based diets, and multi-target compounds like polyphenols are so effective, and even why certain diseases (e.g., autoimmune diseases) are considered incurable from a reductionistic Western medical perspective paradigm. Curing a complex dysregulation inherently requires a multi-pronged strategy.

It's early enough in the process of defining how redox imbalance should be treated that I would not claim to be delivering definitive cures for incurable diseases. Nevertheless, I think the science has progressed to where we can begin to understand and demonstrate why multi-prong treatment approaches are necessary. So paradoxically, the simplicity of redox imbalance causing disease becomes complicated over time because oxidative damage and redox dysregulation potentially affect every downstream system by a bewildering array of mechanisms that we are at the very beginning of understanding despite enormous progress over the last two decades.

The Science Behind Emerging Redox Health Therapies

Despite the absence of established protocols for the treatment of redox imbalance in western medicine, there is a surprisingly robust body of research into how diseases work and how various phytochemicals, vitamins, minerals, amino acids, and botanicals with long histories of medical use provide benefits. This research is well-aligned with a redox health paradigm even though the impetus for this research appears to be largely drug discovery.

I also need to acknowledge that formulating and attempting to flesh out a new treatment paradigm for human disease is an undertaking so vast, complicated, and interconnected that I can only point in its general direction and give outlines and snippets of information on things that have good research support for working. I realize that this leaves me open to all sorts of criticism that I am doing something dangerous and even irresponsible. That critique has some validity, but what keeps me moving forward is the realization that the one thing more dangerous and irresponsible than attempting to build a new treatment paradigm is clinging to an outdated one.

Interpreting the Research for a New Paradigm: A Tall Task

It may be most helpful to begin by giving examples of challenges I've faced in parsing the science while conceptualizing this alternate treatment paradigm:

Omission and Focus

A scientist must necessarily focus their attention on a hypothesis and provide evidence supporting or failing to support it. Thus, a scientist studying the interrelationship of the HPA axis, sympathetic nervous system, and immune system may never mention the renin-angiotensin-aldosterone system, but that doesn't mean that it's not activated along with systems being studied. (It is.) Similarly, a study that shows that HPA axis activation causes cellular oxidative stress may not deal with whether the reverse is true—that oxidative stress causes HPA axis activation. (It does.) To get the full picture of what's going on, you have to read many studies from many different perspectives and make inferences—lots of inferences. You are, in effect, building a mosaic where many of the pieces are missing, and each piece, each fact, drawn from disparate sources, makes the picture clearer.

Not Everything Is Relevant

A couple of years ago, I discussed the applicability of microRNA research to my exploration of redox imbalance with a friend/research scientist. His assessment was that microRNA research, while interesting, had a difficult path to clinical application because a single microRNA might have a hundred different targets in the cell. Thus, it would be hard to make a microRNA therapy that didn't have unwanted side effects. Scientific research is often purely about discovery, with no expectation of practical application. It is then up to the reader to judge the applicability and relevance of any given discovery.

Similarly, many studies are designed out of the values of the current medical paradigm that, while interesting, are simply not where I want to expend energy. A good example of this is studies of immunosuppression/TNFα inhibitors. These drugs, while not totally without value, are a textbook example of Western medicine intervening at the symptom level and not addressing root cause issues, with predictable subpar outcomes at great cost. I don't totally ignore these studies, but neither do I spend a lot of time on them. I want to know why the immune system is chronically activated. It is most likely due to sterile inflammation, a hidden or chronic low-grade infection or intestinal permeability, and downstream endotoxemia.

Translating Paradigms

I am reading research through the lens of the redox imbalance treatment paradigm. That research was primarily written from the perspective of the current Western medical paradigm. That necessarily means that some level of translation is going on, and while I try to get that right, I'm sure that sometimes I miss the mark.

Research Gaps and Differing Priorities

A redox imbalance treatment paradigm's research priorities are undeniably different from those of the current medical paradigm. It's no exaggeration to say that I'm writing this book because redox imbalance has been hiding in plain sight as a root cause of disease, and we do not measure, diagnose, or treat it. That deserves to be studied, and in a redox health paradigm, it would be. There are many other examples of these gaps, and frankly, I don't think they'd be all that hard to fill. They include

- Proving that oxidative stress causes intracellular magnesium deficiency. There is plenty of evidence that it does, but it needs to be conclusively demonstrated and widely acknowledged.
- Identifying other oxidative stress-driven nutritional deficiencies and drawing a much clearer picture of the underlying mechanisms of their depletion. Studies of sepsis give us a good picture of what's happening, but again, it needs to be conclusively demonstrated and widely acknowledged.
- Demonstrating that a significant portion of the impact of infections is oxidative stress-related, whether from direct

pathogenic activity or the resulting immune response. Again, there is good evidence that it's true, and if so, it explains why COVID-19 damages the liver, kidneys, heart, vasculature, and brain and why a Zika infection might cause birth defects. It also points to the need to study whether an intervention with N-acetylcysteine or a NRF2 stimulator (to boost glutathione levels) might prevent Zika-induced birth defects or COVID-related comorbidities.

- Demonstrating conclusively that host resilience and immune status can be bolstered. If I had to pick a failing in the public health response to COVID-19, it would be this: a year into the pandemic, there is still not a universal acknowledgment that low host resilience and immune status due to comorbidities and aging were key determinants of the severity of the pandemic and that raising host resilience and immune status is feasible and important. Thus, while we could bring multiple COVID vaccines to market in under a year, we still can't recommend a protocol to prevent severe COVID-19 based on lowering NLR, raising vitamin D status to >40ng/ml, and taking any of several over-the-counter compounds with strong evidence of antiviral effects and immunomodulation (zinc, selenium, N-acetylcysteine, quercetin, curcumin, EGCG, resveratrol, melatonin, naringin, etc.). It is noteworthy that the Institute of Functional Medicine has produced such a protocol, but it is not widely acknowledged beyond Functional Medicine circles.[143]

I could go on, but the point is that paradigms matter not in small part because they influence research and treatment priorities.

---

143 The Functional Medicine Approach to COVID-19: Virus-Specific Nutraceutical and Botanical Agents

Redox Health Therapies: Reducing Reliance on Prescription Pills and Procedures

Despite the recurring popular press articles warning against non-prescription therapies, many of the compounds being studied as drug discovery candidates are effective enough to use therapeutically. They are also largely over-the-counter and relatively inexpensive compared to prescription drugs and often come with fewer side effects than their prescription counterparts. Redox therapies employing these compounds are based on several foundational assumptions:

- The body has innate abilities to heal once the oxidative stressor is removed or reduced or resilience is increased
- Heightened reactivity/sensitivity (allergies, hives, swelling, skin conditions, etc.) is a sign of redox imbalance and particularly depleted antioxidant capacity, specifically depleted glutathione levels. Glutathione is a key immune-regulating compound that specifically inhibits NF-κB activation, inflammasome activation, and antibody-mediated activation of the classic immune complement system. The immune complement system is like an overdrive mode for the immune system. Thus, you can think of low intracellular glutathione (GSH) as a scenario that invites a hyperreactive immune response to an ordinary immune challenge.[144]
- Fighting oxidative stress raises nutritional demands on key minerals, vitamins, enzymes, and amino acids, and these may require supplementation or dietary shifts to restore proper status. These nutritional deficits are more predictable than currently acknowledged.
- Identifying the sources of ongoing oxidative stress and reduced antioxidant capacity is an important diagnostic imperative. The most common sources are:

---

144 Zhang, Zhen et al. "Glutathione inhibits antibody and complement-mediated immunologic cell injury via multiple mechanisms." *Redox biology* vol. 12 (2017): 571-581. doi:10.1016/j.redox.2017.03.030

- Dietary: processed carbs, sugar, grain oils, dairy, food additives and preservatives, overconsumption of meat, particularly beef and processed meats, high heat cooking, and associated compounds (e.g., AGEs, acrylamides, hydroxynonenal)
  - Too little or too much sleep, or poor sleep quality
  - Inactivity
  - Infection
  - Relational and work stress
  - Prescription and over-the-counter medications (e.g., NSAIDs, PPIs, antibiotics)
  - Recreational drugs and alcohol
  - Environmental toxins
  - Low nutritional status
  - Intestinal permeability
  - Vascular permeability, including blood-brain barrier permeability
  - Gut dysbiosis
  - Poor oral health
  - Physical misalignments/malfunctions
  - Immune system dysregulation
  - Chronic activation of the immune system, HPA axis, renin-angiotensin-aldosterone system, and sympathetic nervous system
- Restoring redox balance, antioxidant capacity, and addressing nutritional status are key therapeutic goals.
- If you don't need it, it won't help you.
- If you get too much, it could hurt you.
- Whole, nutrient-dense, minimally-processed foods are the preferred nutritional maintenance strategy.
- Supplementation can work as a health intervention, and in advanced cases, may be an ongoing necessity. This is particularly true in aging, which is a redox-driven disease with multiple known and addressable pathologies (e.g., low glutathione and NAD+ status)
- The bioavailability of supplements is an issue. Just because you take it doesn't mean you absorb it. Supplement quality and formulation matter.

- Genetic differences play an important role in both symptom presentation and treatment options and efficacy.
- Measuring nutrient status is optimal. Treating symptoms of nutrient deficiency, though less precise, can still work.
- Understanding your genetic profile is increasingly useful. To give one concrete example, G6PD deficiency is a genetically-driven condition that affects 1 in 10 people of African descent but only 1 in 100 whites. People with G6PD deficiency are more vulnerable to oxidative stress and more likely to suffer from glutathione depletion. Thus, G6PD deficiency has been proposed as an explanation for higher COVID-19 death rates among African-Americans.[145] Knowing this has ramifications for understanding risk and potentially how we treat patients with this genetic condition.
- Research into the role of genetics in disease is ongoing. As a rule, maintaining healthy redox status helps prevent undesirable genes from getting "switched on."

With this collection of *a priori* assumptions, we will begin to explore the new Redox treatment paradigm through the lens of the doctor–patient relationship.

Envisioning a Redox Treatment Paradigm: Reimagining the Doctor-Patient Relationship

As a researcher and health consumer, I am keenly aware of the importance of the doctor-patient relationship and its potential to go awry, leaving everyone frustrated. As I've thought about how a redox-centric health paradigm might affect both treatment and prevention of disease, viewing that change through the lens of the doctor–patient relationship seems to

---

[145] Buinitskaya, Yuliya et al. "Centrality of G6PD in COVID-19: The Biochemical Rationale and Clinical Implications." *Frontiers in medicine* vol. 7 584112. 22 Oct. 2020, doi:10.3389/fmed.2020.584112

be a good strategy for making a lot of complex information tangible.

Reimagining the Doctor-Patient Relationship: Exploring the Genome and Exposome Together

When you see a new doctor, there's an obligatory health history that you fill out in the waiting room. These are generally not standardized and are typically dependent on the patient's memory and detail orientation for accuracy and completeness. The sequencing of the human genome in 2001 and the arrival of low-cost DNA sequencing holds significant promise for providing patients and doctors with useful, objective information about a person's genetic makeup and its ramifications for current and future health issues.

Despite initial optimism, researchers and clinicians have had to admit that only a small percentage of diseases were actually directly caused by genetic factors alone. This realization led to the concept of the exposome, which can be understood as the sum total of environmental health-related exposures from conception onward, and perhaps even in the lives of previous generations. The exposome is to epigenetics what the genome is to genetics.

The motivation behind detailing a person's exposome is the realization that early life experiences have lifelong health impacts. Examples of this include fetal alcohol syndrome, prenatal maternal smoking or drug use, shaken baby syndrome, vaginal birth versus C-section, breastfeeding versus bottle feeding, preschool, other mental enrichment activities, reading versus TV watching, earaches, and early antibiotic use, lead paint exposure. Furthermore, health-related exposures throughout life can precipitate health crises and chronic health problems—a junk food diet, an accident, a tick bite, a food poisoning incident, alcoholism, working the night shift, the death of a child, a divorce—these and a million other possible exposures, known and unknown, can shape your healthspan and lifespan.

Treating Redox Imbalance

In a redox treatment paradigm, the doctor-patient relationship is significantly about the following:

- Exploring the interrelationship of the patient's genome and exposome to understand their risk profile.
- Using learnings from redox biology research to identify and mitigate the genetic risks and eliminate or mitigate the patients' stressors.
- Bolstering antioxidant capacity, nutritional status, and stress-resilience to resolve or mitigate any associated damage and dysregulation.
- Identifying pro-inflammatory states and feed-forward loops that are sustaining the redox imbalance and addressing them.

Detailing the individual patient's exposome is a combination of a good health history instrument and electronic medical record system, bolstered by public health data about generalizable health-related measures—e.g., regional air quality, water quality and mineral content, fluoridation, and socioeconomic data down to the neighborhood level. There are large-scale public health infrastructure ramifications implied here, but fortunately, this is an agenda that others are already pursuing. While it's not my purpose to build a new health history/exposome survey here, I would envision it gathering information such as:

Pre-birth
- Did your mother receive prenatal care during her pregnancy?
- Did your mother smoke, drink or use drugs during her pregnancy?
- Did your mother have any significant health challenges during her pregnancy?
- Were you born by C-section?
- Were you breastfed or bottle-fed?
- Were you born prematurely?
- Did you feel wanted as a child?

Early childhood
- Were you adopted? If so, at what age?
- Did you receive your vaccinations according to the recommended schedule?
- Did you have recurrent earaches before the age of three?
- Did you receive antibiotics, to your knowledge?
- Did you participate in preschool or a Head Start program?
- How would you characterize your height and weight as a child? Above Average –> Average –> Below Average?
- While growing up, would you describe your family's diet as healthy or unhealthy?
- Which best describes where you grew up? A large city, small city, suburb, rural, farm
- Did you have any outstanding health issues as a child?
- Did you experience anything as a child that you would describe as trauma, either psychological or physical?

Adolescence
- List your age of first experience and frequency of the following:
  - Drug and alcohol use
  - Sex
  - Smartphone use
  - Social media use
- In a given week, how many times did you eat/drink the following (0–7x):
  - Sweetened breakfast cereal
  - Dessert
  - Fried food
  - Grilled food
  - Fast food
  - Soft drinks
  - Alcohol
- List any medications you took as a teen.
- List any medical issues you experienced as a teen.
- Did you experience anything as a teen that you would describe as trauma, either psychological or physical?

Adulthood
- <standard health history questions>
- Rate the stress level of your workplace.
- Rate the stress level of your home life.
- I have trouble sleeping. Never –> frequently
- I experience anxiety or depression. Never –> frequently
- I work around toxic chemicals or cleaning supplies. Never –> frequently
- In a given week, how many times do you eat/drink the following (0–7x):
  - Sweetened breakfast cereal
  - Dessert
  - Fried food
  - Grilled food
  - Fast food
  - Soft drinks
  - Alcohol
- Did you experience anything as an adult that you would describe as trauma, either psychological or physical?
- What medications do you take?
- What supplements do you take?
- How would you characterize your diet? Vegetarian, Vegan, Pescatarian, Omnivore, Paleo, Other.

The initial testing workup would include
- Standard health biomarkers—weight, waist/height ratio, blood pressure, fasting glucose/HbA1c, resting heart rate, heart rate variability, homocysteine levels, etc.
- A complete blood count and calculation of neutrophil/lymphocyte ratio (NLR) as the "good enough" surrogate for redox imbalance and stress resilience.
- Testing for nutritional status—are you deficient in key vitamins, minerals, and amino acids?
- Testing for redox status—Thiol/disulfide ratio, malondialdehyde, f2-isoprostanes, protein carbonyls, TAC, TOS, etc.). *Note: there's a reasonable case to be made that these tests should be done after determining that NLR is elevated, particularly if testing costs remain high.*

- Testing for infection—do you have active and/or low-grade chronic infections?
- Testing for barrier function/health—e.g., lactulose/mannitol testing, serum zonulin, and iFABP levels. *Note: at the time of this writing, there is controversy over the accuracy of serum zonulin tests.*
- Checking for misalignments: one leg longer than the other, one shoulder higher than the other, curvature of the spine, damage to the spine or neck vertebra, signs of injury or trauma, etc.

Caveat: This kind of testing is not standardized and is thus subject to refinement, trust-building, and cost reduction on the way to broader clinical usage and patient benefit.

Early doctor-patient sessions would entail going over the genome, exposome, and initial testing and its relation to any current symptoms or conditions. Symptoms are grouped based on where they fall under any of the following redox pathologies:

- Cellular redox imbalance and downstream dysregulation, including
  - Mitochondrial damage/dysfunction
  - Endoplasmic reticulum stress/proteome dysregulation
  - DNA Damage in the nucleus or mitochondria
  - Calcium loading/calcium channel dysregulation
  - Insulin resistance/glucose intolerance
  - Cell life cycle dysregulation affecting:
    - Angiogenesis
    - Mutagenesis
    - Apoptosis
    - Necrosis
    - Replication
    - Autophagy
    - Senescence
- Chronic HPA axis activation/dysregulation

- Chronic renin-angiotensin-aldosterone system activation/dysregulation
- Low/dysregulated nutritional status
- Chronic sympathetic nervous system activation/sympathetic-parasympathetic imbalance
- Chronic immune system activation/dysregulation
- Intestinal permeability
- Gut dysbiosis
- Vascular permeability/endothelial dysfunction
- Physical stressors
- Genetic/epigenetic stress and signaling dysregulation

The above pathologies are the pathways of most chronic disease. By the time you are symptomatic, typically, multiple pathologies are involved. One of the advantages of this approach is the speed of diagnosis and early intervention. On patient forums, one of the recurring complaints is, "My doctors can't figure out what's wrong with me—still waiting for a diagnosis." Since diagnosis precedes the assignment of a treatment protocol, meaningful intervention is delayed. In the above approach, you identify which pathologies and relevant feedforward mechanisms are involved and treat each of them. Often, this alone will be sufficient to resolve the symptoms, as your body's homeostatic mechanisms are unblocked and allowed to resolve the root cause issues.

As doctor and patient explore the genome–exposome interaction, the conversation quickly turns to diet and lifestyle issues. Many doctors complain that patients don't want to change their diet and lifestyle. They just want a pill, and in more extreme cases, they want a procedure to fix whatever is wrong. While that may be true in many cases, it is largely a situation created by the medical/pharmaceutical industry and broader society. Collectively, we have created an anti-health culture and a medical-industrial complex designed to monitor you as your high-stress, low-nutrient, high-toxicity lifestyle degrades your health and quality of life. Then that self-same system manages your chronic diseases as you acquire them, often from the prescribed medications' side effects.

While this is a much bigger problem than any individual doctor can tackle, the moral obligation of the healthcare provider is to point patients away from lifestyle choices that are anti-health and toward things that are pro-health, particularly things that are within the patient's control. Medical science is giving us a much clearer picture of what those things are, and they start with diet and lifestyle issues, such as sleep, inactivity, and psychological stress.

Reimagining the Doctor-Patient Relationship: A Conversation about Resilience Habits

In the last chapter, we detailed various resilience habits that health consumers can explore to enhance their resilience to future mental and physical stress. While most of these practices are currently viewed as outside the domain of western clinical practice, the idea that your doctor would be a partner in optimizing your resilience habits would be game-changing. There are precedents for this happening, mostly in the realm of diet, where a growing group of "veggie docs" are amassing thousands of patient stories of disease reversal, reduction or elimination of the need for prescription medicine, weight loss, avoidance of heart surgery and massive improvements to overall health and well-being. They include doctors Caldwell Esselstyn, James McDougall, Joel Fuhrman, Dean Ornish, and many others.

While their advocacy for the health benefits of plant-based eating has been incredibly important and useful, my purpose in promoting understanding of redox imbalance is to build and expand on that foundation to include and interconnect the entire span of resilience practices. In the last chapter, we saw how the various resilience habits shared common biological pathways—NRF2, AMPK, SIRT1, FOXO, PGC1a—conferring resilience to future stress through a broad range of epigenetic adaptations. How you stimulate these pathways, whether through diet, exercise, heat/cold exposure, dietary supplements (e.g., polyphenols), prescription meds (e.g., metformin, statins), calorie restriction/fasting, vagus nerve stimulation, the effects of that stimulation varies with the mode. Thus, it seems logical that we would cultivate a broad collection of synergistic resilience habits, and our doctors would be partners in optimizing our strategies and monitoring our progress. This is obviously a vision for a future that does not yet exist, but hey, let's run with it.

Imagine a future where you've authorized your doctor's medical practice to receive health data from your smartwatch/phone. You, of course, have the right to limit access to certain kinds of data if you choose, and your doctor has let you know what kind of information is useful to her. At your annual physical, your doctor pulls up your wellness and resilience progress report and notes the following:

- You closed your rings on 86% of the days since your last check-up, which is good, but your overall activity is trending down over the last six months. Anything going on that would be contributing to that?
- Since starting your fitness training program, your average mile time has dropped from 14 minutes to under 10 minutes, which is good progress.
- Your heart rate variability is still below the median for someone your age. Your doctor recommends that you increase your yoga workouts' number and duration and perhaps add some 4:8:8 breathing to your resilience practices.
- Your blood pressure averaged 132/86 over the last two weeks, another sign of sympathovagal imbalance. She notes that upping your yoga and deep breathing may be sufficient to get that in the normal range, but we'll want to be watching that.
- Your triglyceride levels are up from 150 to 190, which is indicative of eating more carbs and sugar, so you might want to cut back.
- Your average sleep time is 6.5 hours per night, and your doctor asks if that feels about right. She notes that she sees several nighttime blood oxygenation drops below 90%, which can indicate sleep apnea. She recommends an

appointment with the sleep specialist to get to the bottom of that since sleep apnea is a significant contributor to heart disease and early death.
- Your neutrophil/lymphocyte ratio is 1.8, down from 2.0 last physical, which is good progress. Less inflammation = less oxidative stress and more resilience. Pat yourself on the back!

Frankly, that conversation could happen based on technology that is available today. I could have thrown in genetic profiling, metabolomic blood scans, personalized nutrition recommendations, and AI-driven analysis of hundreds or even thousands of biomarkers.

Reimagining the Doctor-Patient Relationship: A Conversation about Nutrition

While nutrient-dense eating is a core resilience strategy for supplying your body with the nutrients it needs for proper function, nutrition deserves its own dedicated conversation as an undervalued intervention in a variety of chronic and acute diseases and symptoms. Advances in the understanding and treatment of critical illness (e.g., sepsis and COVID-19) and trauma have highlighted both the role of malnutrition in these conditions and the importance of addressing these nutritional deficits in preventing death and promoting recovery.

Accumulating evidence shows that redox status, immune status, and nutritional status are interwoven to the point that they are at times practically indistinguishable. Examples of this include
- Glutathione is your body's primary antioxidant. It also plays both functional and regulatory roles in the immune system, inhibiting viral replication and regulating innate immunity and inflammation through redox signaling. Depletion of glutathione is recognized as weakening the immune response in several infectious diseases.
- Glutathione's precursors are amino acids, and the cofactors

necessary for glutathione production and recycling are largely vitamins and minerals.
- The COVID-19 pandemic, like battlefield medicine, allowed us to witness death by COVID-19 and comorbid sepsis. It was routinely accompanied by malnutrition (low nutritional status), low redox status (elevated ROS/diminished GSH), and lowered immune status and dysregulation (the cytokine storm) that resulted in multiple organ failure and death. While it currently falls in the realm of medical hypothesis, I consider it highly likely that these three interrelated phenomena are both the cause of COVID mortality and hold the key to more effective COVID treatments.

The key principle here is that nutritional interventions, along with your resilience habits, are highly desirable strategies because they are inexpensive, low risk, and have minimal side effects. Furthermore, stress-driven nutritional deficits are often root cause issues in the symptoms and diseases we are trying to treat, and that can make them very effective.

This, of course, is not how medical protocols currently work, yet there are signs that this is changing. In May 2020, the US National Institutes of Health (NIH) announced a 10-year strategic plan to speed up nutritional research, with goal of achieving precision nutrition—where we each have individualized recommendations that help us decide "what, when, why, and how to eat to optimize our health and quality of life."[146] The plan has four strategic goals:

1. Spur Discovery and Innovation through Foundational Research: What do we eat and how does it affect us?
2. Investigate the Role of Dietary Patterns and Behaviors for Optimal Health: What and when should we eat?
3. Define the Role of Nutrition Across the Lifespan: How does what we eat promote health across our lifespan?
4. Reduce the Burden of Disease in Clinical Settings: How can we improve the use of food as medicine?

---

146 2020-2030 Strategic Plan for NIH Nutrition Research

Having the NIH getting behind nutritional research and precision nutrition in this way is potentially game-changing. It also represents just the latest step in a journey towards recognizing the importance of nutrition in health and healthcare and how it intersects with the broader goals of precision medicine.

Triggers for the Conversation

The doctor-patient conversation about nutrition could be triggered by a rising neutrophil/lymphocyte ratio (NLR), other inflammatory biomarkers, weight gain (or loss), a cardiovascular biomarker that is trending in the wrong direction (i.e., resting heart rate, heart rate variability or blood pressure), or some other health complaint or disease symptom.

Key components of that conversation would include

Minimize Nutritional Stressors

The key sources of nutritional stress and inflammation in the western diet are refined carbohydrates, sugar, grain oils, food additives and preservatives, and over-consumption of animal products, particularly beef and processed meats. Beyond these, there are food sensitivities such as gluten, lectin and lactose intolerance, and nut allergies resulting in inflammatory responses. The sensitivities are highly individual, and the response can vary over time, even for the same person. If your NLR or other inflammatory markers are elevated, this step is mandatory and can yield a significant reduction in symptoms.

Bolster Redox Status

While stress causes redox imbalance, part of the mechanism at work is the depletion of key nutrients involved in maintaining redox status. Because redox imbalance plays a role in every downstream disease and depleted glutathione status is a component of critical illness, aging, and chronic illness, understanding and addressing these nutritional deficits should be a foundational strategy for treating any disease, with the possible exception of active cancer where glutathione and NRF2 activation can play a role in tumor growth and protection of tumor cells from excess ROS and immune system processes designed to destroy such cells. Nutritional players in raising glutathione include

- **Glutathione Precursors**. All three of the following amino acids are considered rate-limiting for glutathione production:
  - L-glutamine is converted to glutamic acid, a glutathione precursor. It can be depleted in exercise, and cellular glutamine deprivation has been shown to raise oxidative stress levels. Supplementation with L-glutamine to raise glutathione has shown mixed results, suggesting that in the absence of a glutamine deficit, excess L-glutamine can actually interfere with glutathione production.
  - Cysteine, typically derived from animal and plant protein sources, can be depleted in high-demand situations, such as critical illness. Supplementally, cysteine can be delivered through N-acetylcysteine and other sulfur amino acids (e.g., taurine) or whey protein.
  - Glycine is an amino acid that is sweet and looks and measures like sugar. Supplementation with glycine has been shown to raise tissue GSH and improve the GSH/GSSG ratio.
- **Glutathione Cofactors**
  - Vitamins B1, thiamine is essential for glutathione recycling.
  - B2, riboflavin, is a coenzyme for glutathione reductase, which participates in glutathione synthesis
  - B6, pyridoxine, promotes glutathione synthesis through homocysteine > cysteine conversion and transsulfuration of proteins for the glutathione peroxidase system. In the brain, pyridoxine facilitates GSH synthesis via the PKM2-Nrf2 pathway.[147]

---

[147] Wei, Y., Lu, M., Mei, M. *et al.* "Pyridoxine induces glutathione synthesis via PKM2-mediated Nrf2 transactivation and confers neuroprotection.". *Nat Commun* 11, 941 (2020). doi.org/10.1038/s41467-020-14788-x.

- B9, folate, regulates the synthesis of glutathione via modulation of GSH/GSSG and NADPH/NADP+ redox couples.[148]
- B12, cobalamin, deficiency blocks the conversion of homocysteine to cysteine, limiting glutathione synthesis.
- Vitamin C (ascorbate) intake correlates with glutathione and total antioxidant status.[149] Supplementation with 500 mg of vitamin C raised red blood cell glutathione in study subjects, and higher doses did not make significant improvements.[150]
- Vitamin D3 upregulates glutamyl-cysteine ligase, an enzyme that catalyzes glutathione synthesis.[151]
- Vitamin E, a tocopherol, as an antioxidant, participates in the recycling of GSSG to GSH.
- Minerals magnesium, selenium, and zinc. These antioxidant minerals all participate in the synthesis and recycling of glutathione. Magnesium increases glutathione peroxidase activity. Zinc deficiency negatively affects γ-Glutamylcysteine, the first enzyme in the glutathione synthesis pathway.
- a-Lipoic acid

- **NRF2 stimulators** and the epigenetic upregulation of glutathione and 200+ other stress resilience-related genes.
  - Phytonutrients quercetin, rutin, curcumin, berberine, pterostilbene, sulforaphane, resveratrol, EGCG and others.

---

148 Lai, Kun-Goung, et al. "Novel Roles of Folic Acid as Redox Regulator: Modulation of Reactive Oxygen Species Sinker Protein Expression and Maintenance of Mitochondrial Redox Homeostasis on Hepatocellular Carcinoma." *Tumor Biology*, June 2017, doi:10.1177/1010428317702649.

149 Waly, Mostafa I et al. "Low Nourishment of Vitamin C Induces Glutathione Depletion and Oxidative Stress in Healthy Young Adults." *Preventive nutrition and food science* vol. 20,3 (2015): 198-203. doi:10.3746/pnf.2015.20.3.198

150 Johnston, C S et al. "Vitamin C elevates red blood cell glutathione in healthy adults." *The American journal of clinical nutrition* vol. 58,1 (1993): 103-5. doi:10.1093/ajcn/58.1.103

151 Singh, Mohkam et al. "Understanding the Relationship between Glutathione, TGF-β, and Vitamin D in Combating *Mycobacterium tuberculosis* Infections." *Journal of clinical medicine* vol. 9,9 2757. 26 Aug. 2020, doi:10.3390/jcm9092757

- **NAD+ precursors**/regulators
  - Nicotinamide Riboside, Nicotinamide Mononucleotide
  - Taurine[152]

Focus on Nutrient Quality and Density

When dietitians talk about the six essential nutrients, they are referring to proteins, carbohydrates, fats, water, vitamins, and minerals. If you like endless debates on dietary philosophies, focus on macronutrients (proteins, fats, and carbohydrates) and their optimal ratio in your diet. Much of the historical debate has been over high protein/low protein diets, high fat/low-fat diets, and high carbohydrate/low carbohydrate diets. The failure of this approach is evident in the US health statistics:

- Obesity rate: 42.4%, up from 30.5% in 2000.[153]
- Diabetes rate (total diagnosed and undiagnosed): 13% (2016), up from 9.5% in 2000.[154]
- Over six million Americans have Alzheimer's disease. Alzheimer's disease deaths are up 145% since 2000.[155]
- Six in 10 adults have a chronic disease. Four in 10 have two or more.[156]
- Cancer rates are largely flat thanks to decreased smoking rates, though an estimated 1.8 million Americans will be diagnosed with cancer in 2020.[157]
- Heart disease rates are also largely flat, but the disease is nonetheless considered an epidemic that affects over 125

---

152 Jing Liu, Yongfei Ai, Xiaolin Niu, Fujun Shang, Zhili Li, Hui Liu, Wei Li, Wenshuai Ma, Ruirui Chen, Ting Wei, Xue Li, Xiaoli Li. "Taurine protects against cardiac dysfunction induced by pressure overload through SIRT1–p53 activation." Chemico-Biological Interactions, Volume 317, 2020, 108972, ISSN 0009-2797, doi.org/10.1016/j.cbi.2020.108972.

153 "Adult Obesity Facts." https://www.cdc.gov/obesity/data/adult.html

154 "Diabetes Statistics Report, 2020" https://www.cdc.gov/diabetes/pdfs/data/statistics/national-diabetes-statistics-report.pdf

155 "Alzheimers and Dementia Facts and Figures." https://www.alz.org/alzheimers-dementia/facts-figures

156 "Chronic Diseases in America" https://www.cdc.gov/chronicdisease/resources/infographic/chronic-diseases.htm

157 "Cancer Statistics." https://www.cancer.gov/about-cancer/understanding/statistics

million Americans and accounts for 42.1% of all deaths (2018 data).[158]

If there was an employee in charge of those outcomes, they'd already be fired.

To illustrate the failure of the macronutrient nutrient approach, I offer my own experience as a patient:

> *Back in 2011, I, as a newly-minted type 2 diabetic (HbA1C = 6.3), attended my local hospital's nutrition training for diabetics, and it was very macronutrient focused: 1 protein choice, 1 carb choice, 2 non-starchy vegetables, a side of fruit and a glass of milk. Despite being pretty unsophisticated at that point, I asked if we would talk about carbohydrate quality and was told no. I really wanted to cure my diabetes rather than manage it, so I went home and started looking for answers elsewhere. Note that "The Healthy Diabetes Plate" was developed at the University of Idaho in the early 2000s and continues to be the gold standard diabetes training for managing type 2 diabetes. While there are undeniably some virtues in keeping it simple, what they fail to tell you is that the cure for type 2 diabetes and many other chronic illnesses lies at the micronutrient level, where 30+ essential vitamins and minerals and literally thousands of phytonutrients reduce oxidative stress and inflammation, reverse insulin resistance, keep blood vessels healthy, balance systems, regulate and bolster immune function and a host of other health-inducing actions.*

Focusing on nutrient density works because it steers you away from the processed food aisles and cooking oils (calorie-dense) and towards leafy greens, fruits and vegetables, nuts, seeds, legumes/pulses, mushrooms, herbs, and spices. Meat and fish aren't off-limits, but neither are they the central focus

---

158 "2021 Heart Disease and Stroke Statistics Update Fact Sheet." https://www.heart.org/-/media/phd-files-2/science-news/2/2021-heart-and-stroke-stat-update/2021_heart_disease_and_stroke_statistics_update_fact_sheet_at_a_glance.pdf

of meal planning. Aphorisms such as "If you can't pronounce the ingredients, don't buy it," or even, "If it has a label, don't buy it," can be useful guides as long as you don't turn them into laws.

Focusing on nutrient quality works because it steers you away from the western food industry's worst sins: refined carbohydrates and sugar, artificial sweeteners, grains oils, unhealthy additives (soybean oil, high fructose corn syrup, dough conditioners, artificial colors, sweeteners, preservatives, etc.). The definition of processed foods expands from refined carbohydrates to include most dairy products (pasteurized, homogenized) and even things you wouldn't suspect, such as commercial orange juice.

Learn About Immunonutrients

While the idea that vitamins and minerals played a role in immune function has been around since the early 20th century, immunonutrition as a term first appears in the scientific literature in the 1980s in relation to cancer patients getting prepped for bowel surgery. Doctors noted that albumin, prealbumin, and lymphocyte levels, biomarkers of malnutrition were lower in the cancer patients. Immunonutrition becomes associated with enteral/parenteral feeding (feeding by tube) of surgical patients and the critically ill in the '90s with a relatively narrow set of nutrients with known immunologic function.

Nearly thirty years later, the immunonutrition field has evolved and begun to consider a much broader range of nutrients and strategies to combat the immune-inflammatory health effects stemming from the global spread of the western diet—obesity, diabetes, cardiovascular disease, cancer, neurodegenerative diseases, and other chronic and autoimmune diseases.[159] While there is more detail in nutrition

---

[159] Magrone Thea, Haslberger Alexander, Jirillo Emilio, Serafini Mauro. "Editorial: Immunonutrient Supplementation." Frontiers in Nutrition, Vol. 6 2019, doi:10.3389/fnut.2019.00182

research than anyone can master and much yet to be learned and proven, several principles are coming into view. These principles are a useful starting point for patients. They include

1. Critical, acute, and chronic illness and other stressors cause immunonutrient deficiencies that are potentially correctable through diet, supplementation, and enteral nutrition.
2. Dysregulations of the immune system, including allergy, low immunity, and autoimmunity, can be ameliorated or reversed via nutritional interventions.
3. Immune status, redox status, and nutritional status are intertwined to the point of inseparability. Stressors impact all three.
4. A recent review of micronutrients that support healthy immune function included: vitamins A, D, C, E, B6, B12, folate, copper, iron, zinc, and selenium, with the bulk of research to date focusing on Vitamin C, Vitamin D3, and Zinc.[160] When you include phytonutrients, the number of potentially useful compounds jumps into the thousands.
5. Malnutrition can cause disease. Correct nutrition can cure disease. With its abundance of low-nutrient calorie-dense, highly-processed foods, the western diet is a cause of malnutrition.
6. Immune system function extends beyond clearing pathogens to include wound healing, cell and tissue damage repair, detoxification, clearance of dead, damaged, senescent and mutated cells.
7. Chronic activation of the immune system by pathogens, cellular damage, toxins, and other stressors produce inflammation (sterile and pathogenic) that contributes to a broad range of chronic diseases. Redox systems are critical regulators of the inflammatory process.[161]
8. Abuse of antibiotics and the rise of antibiotic-resistant

---

160 Derbyshire, Emma, and Joanne Delange. "COVID-19: is there a role for immunonutrition, particularly in the over 65s?." *BMJ nutrition, prevention & health* vol. 3,1 100-105. 16 Apr. 2020, doi:10.1136/bmjnph-2020-000071

161 Singla, Bhupesh et al. "Editorial: Oxidants and Redox Signaling in Inflammation." *Frontiers in immunology* vol. 10 545. 26 Mar. 2019, doi:10.3389/fimmu.2019.00545

bacteria have led to increased research into alternative strategies, including antimicrobial peptides and antimicrobial plant compounds. Many of these compounds are effective against not only bacteria, but viruses, fungi, parasites and even some cancers.

Caveats: This list is my own, and I acknowledge that it would be controversial in a medical setting despite accumulating evidence to back up the individual principles. Nutritional intervention, like medicine, has instances where it works really well and other instances where it is ineffective or even damaging. Getting to the point where the science is settled and we know definitively what works when, for whom and under what circumstances, will take time. This aligns with the NIH ten-year strategic plan to move towards precision nutrition. I've adopted these principles for my own health and nutrition and believe that they have enhanced my immune status and overall health.

Examples of Immunonutrients

While an exhaustive treatment of each principle is beyond the scope of this book, below are examples of studies and useful applications of immunonutrients:

Zinc. Zinc is one of the most prominent immunonutrients. Zinc deficiency is common, affecting an estimated 2 billion people worldwide. Zinc deficiency significantly impairs immune function, lowering B lymphocyte and T lymphocyte counts, granulocyte and natural killer cell counts, and decreasing phagocytosis by macrophages. This leaves the affected person more vulnerable to not only communicable diseases but also cancer. Zinc is depleted by stress and conditions such as diabetes. Zinc supplementation improves not only immune status, but insulin resistance and glucose production in overweight patients increases GSH and total antioxidant capacity, reduces oxidative damage (e.g., malondialdehyde levels).

Vitamin D. Vitamin D has received lots of attention as an immunonutrient over the course of the COVID-19 pandemic, thanks to the early realization that low vitamin D status was significantly correlated with COVID severity and mortality. More recent studies have shown that 80% of COVID-19 patients were vitamin D deficient. Furthermore, a University of Chicago Study showed black individuals with higher serum vitamin D levels (>40ng/ml) had a 2.64x lower risk of testing positive for COVID than those in the 30-40 ng/ml range. Some countries, including the United Kingdom, are recommending vitamin D supplementation as a COVID-19 prophylactic. One year into the pandemic, evidence that vitamin D3 supplementation reduces COVID-19 mortality and severity is finally beginning to arrive. A 2021 meta-analysis showed decreased mortality rates, reduced severity, and lower inflammation in the vitamin D3 treatment groups but called for more studies to determine the optimal dosage and duration.[162] Beyond COVID, vitamin D supplementation has a long history as a strategy for maintaining bone health (along with vitamin K2, magnesium, and calcium), while more recent attention has focused on its antiviral role in diverse illnesses, including hepatitis, influenza, and AIDS.

Arginine, an amino acid, upregulates nitric oxide synthase, increasing NO production. A 2020 review article found that studies to date support and encourage arginine supplementation in cardiovascular disease, especially for preventing hypertension and atherosclerosis progression.[163]

Glutamine. Glutamine is essential for glutathione synthesis. A low glutamine/glutamate ratio is associated with muscle wasting, reduced immune function, decreased energy, and digestive issues, including intestinal permeability.

---

162 Nikniaz, Leila, et al. "The impact of vitamin D supplementation on mortality rate and clinical outcomes of COVID-19 patients: A systematic review and meta-analysis." medRxiv 2021.01.04.21249219; doi: https://doi.org/10.1101/2021.01.04.21249219

163 Gambardella, Jessica et al. "Arginine and Endothelial Function." *Biomedicines* vol. 8,8 277. 6 Aug. 2020, doi:10.3390/biomedicines8080277

Omega 3 fatty acids. Omega 3 fatty acids promote a healthy microbiome, reduce intestinal permeability and prevent obesity and associated metabolic disorders (in mice). Their reputation for being anti-inflammatory compounds derives from their role as precursors for specific pro-resolving mediators (SPRMs), including defensins, resolvins, and alarmins.

Melatonin. Produced in the pineal gland and gastrointestinal tissue, melatonin is a neurohormone known for regulating circadian rhythms. It is also a potent antioxidant and regulator of immune function. Seasonal fluctuations of melatonin production have been associated with multiple sclerosis relapses. Melatonin supplementation has been studied in multiple sclerosis, where it reduced demyelination, suppressed the Th17 cell population and IL-17 production, and inflammatory compounds IFN-γ, IL-6, and CCL20.[164] Melatonin supplementation also has potential applications in COVID-19 prevention and treatment, cognitive impairment, cardiometabolic diseases. Fish are a good food source for melatonin.

N-acetylcysteine (NAC). In addition to being a glutathione precursor and a first-line therapy for acetaminophen poisoning, NAC thins mucus in the lungs, breaks up bacterial biofilms, reduces infection rates, duration, and severity of the flu, reduces inflammatory and oxidative damage in tissue. NAC has shown benefit in treating diseases including sepsis, lupus, acute liver injury, neuropathy, diabetic nephropathy, COVID-19, anxiety, and depression. In a 2012 randomized clinical trial of lupus patients, N-acetylcysteine showed reliable improvement in standardized assessments for disease activity and severity in under three months and improvements in fatigue scores. Furthermore, the gains

---

164 Yeganeh, Mahshid & Mollica, Adriano & Momtaz, Saeideh & Sanadgol, Nima & Farzaei, Mohammad Hosein. "Melatonin and Multiple Sclerosis: From Plausible Neuropharmacological Mechanisms of Action to Experimental and Clinical Evidence." *Clinical Drug Investigation* vol 39. (2019) doi:10.1007/s40261-019-00793-6.

cost $180-360/year versus $22,580/year for standard, less-effective, side-effect-prone treatments.[165]

Beta glucan. Beta glucans are sugars (polysaccharides) found in various food products, including mushrooms, lichens, algae, bacteria, yeast, and some grains, such as oats and barley. Functionally, they are considered soluble fiber with prebiotic effects. Immunologically, they stimulate macrophage activity and have attracted significant research attention as anticancer/antitumor compounds. As a generalization, cereal beta glucans have glucose and lipid-lowering abilities, while fungal beta glucans have shown greater immunomodulatory traits.[166]

Naringin. Naringin is a flavonoid found in grapefruit skins, with potential therapeutic applications in bone health, cardiometabolic diseases, inflammatory and neurological diseases, and cancer. In a study of flavonoid-related immunomodulation, Naringin inhibited immune-inflammatory cytokines TNF-a and IL-6 in macrophages— IL-6 comparable to quercetin and TNF-a more than quercetin.[167] Supplemental naringin is a key component of grapefruit seed extract.

Learn about Longevity Nutrients

The idea of longevity nutrients comes from a 2018 paper by Bruce Ames. He makes the case that nutrients fall into two classes: survival nutrients necessary for immediate survival and reproduction and longevity nutrients that promote

---

165 Lai, Zhi-Wei et al. "N-acetylcysteine reduces disease activity by blocking mammalian target of rapamycin in T cells from systemic lupus erythematosus patients: a randomized, double-blind, placebo-controlled trial." *Arthritis and rheumatism* vol. 64,9 (2012): 2937-46. doi:10.1002/art.34502

166 Murphy, Emma J et al. "β-Glucan Metabolic and Immunomodulatory Properties and Potential for Clinical Application." *Journal of fungi (Basel, Switzerland)* vol. 6,4 356. 10 Dec. 2020, doi:10.3390/jof6040356

167 Mendes, L.F., Gaspar, V.M., Conde, T.A. *et al.* "Flavonoid-mediated immunomodulation of human macrophages involves key metabolites and metabolic pathways.". *Sci Rep* 9, 14906 (2019). doi.org/10.1038/s41598-019-51113-z

long-term health.[168] The article's importance is perhaps less about his specific list of longevity nutrients than the idea that subclinical nutrient deficiencies promote aging and that we should be looking for nutrients that optimize health and longevity. Ames' list includes
- Vitamin K - deficiency is associated with cardiovascular and all-cause mortality.
- Selenium
- Vitamin D
- Magnesium - Mg intake is inversely associated with all-cause mortality. Low intake was associated with poorer DNA repair capacity and increased lung
- Taurine - upregulates blood levels of hydrogen sulfide (H2S), a regulator of endothelial function, lowering systolic and diastolic BP while improving endothelial function and vasodilation.[169]
- Ergothioneine (ESH)
- Pyrroloquinoline quinone (PQQ).
- Queuine
- Carotenoids
  - Lutein
  - Xeanthin
  - Lycopene
  - a Carotene, b Carotene, B Cryptoxanthin
  - Astaxanthin

To the above list, I would suggest several potential additions:
- Quercetin
- Rutin
- Fisetin is a potent senolytic polyphenol. Testing in mice reduced age-related pathology and increased lifespan

---

168 Ames, Bruce N. "Prolonging healthy aging: Longevity vitamins and proteins." *Proceedings of the National Academy of Sciences of the United States of America* vol. 115,43 (2018): 10836-10844. doi:10.1073/pnas.1809045115

169 Sun, Qianqian et al. "Taurine Supplementation Lowers Blood Pressure and Improves Vascular Function in Prehypertension: Randomized, Double-Blind, Placebo-Controlled Study." *Hypertension (Dallas, Tex. : 1979)* vol. 67,3 (2016): 541-9. doi:10.1161/HYPERTENSIONAHA.115.06624

- Resveratrol
- Berberine

Learn About Probiotics, Prebiotics, and Synbiotics

The digestive tract is perhaps the most undervalued and poorly understood real estate in medicine. Yet its role in maintaining health and homeostasis could hardly be more valuable—the seat of immunity, home to 3 trillion bacterial partners in maintaining health, digesting and absorbing nutrients, and regulating the body's organ systems, the largest collection of neurons and glia outside of the brain (over 100 million!) earning it the title of "the enteric brain." Much of the research on maintaining the digestive tract and microbiome's health has focused on probiotics, prebiotics, and synbiotics, so let's cover the latest science on each.

Probiotics

The idea that consuming beneficial live bacteria could confer health benefits is as old as human civilization. Every culture has examples of fermented, probiotic foods—yogurt, sauerkraut, kombucha, kimchi, kefir, cheese, tempeh, fish sauce, wine, beer, injera, vinegar, and many, many more. The idea that we might do this with pills is very recent (late 20th century) and still controversial given the challenges of delivering sufficient quantities of viable bacteria to the small and large intestines to make a tangible impact. Microbial diversity in the gut microbiome is associated with better health. The threats to that diversity in western culture include a food system that views bacteria as a threat to food transport, safety, shelf life, and ultimately profit. This diet is short on fiber and high in refined carbohydrates and sugars, pharmaceuticals including proton pump inhibitors, laxatives, antibiotics, antidepressants, and antidiabetics that reshape the microbiome constituents. Many of these gut microbiota changes are associated with disease states—obesity, diabetes, liver and neurodegenerative diseases, cancer, and aging. Despite the relative lack of clinical trials in this area, there is reasonable evidence that bacteria from fermented foods reach the microbiome and exert health benefits.[170] Similarly, several probiotic supplement strategies have shown therapeutic efficacy, including

- *Saccharomyces Boulardii* and *Lactobacillus rhamnosus GG* in the treatment of Antibiotic Associated Diarrhea and *Clostridium difficile* infections.
- *Bifidobacterium infantis 35624* in the treatment of irritable bowel syndrome.
- *Bifidobacterium spp.* and *Lactobacillus acidophilus* to prevent necrotizing enterocolitis in low birth weight infants.[171]
- The commercial probiotic mix VSL#3 to reduce intestinal permeability and oxidative stress.[172]

Prebiotics

Increased attention to the role of fiber (soluble and insoluble) and resistant starch in digestive health gave rise to the idea of prebiotics. These dietary substances create a hospitable environment for the growth of desirable bacterial strains with resulting health benefits. The theory and science behind prebiotics help explain the benefits of plant-based diets and specific foods such as beans, peas, lentils, whole grains, Jerusalem artichokes, yams, green bananas, etc., plantain. The primary supplemental prebiotics have been based on inulin fiber, though there is increasing research interest in the prebiotic effects of plant polyphenols, fruit pectins, mushroom beta glucans, and algal polysaccharides. A key benefit of resistant starch and soluble fiber consumption comes from short-chain fatty acids SFCA via their fermentation in the

---

170 Car Reen Kok, Robert Hutkins. "Yogurt and other fermented foods as sources of health-promoting bacteria." *Nutrition Reviews*, Volume 76, Issue Supplement_1, 1 December 2018, Pages 4–15, doi.org/10.1093/nutrit/nuy056

171 Gogineni et al. "Probiotics: History and Evolution." J Anc Dis Prev Rem 2013, 1:2 doi: 10.4172/2329-8731.1000107

172 Cruz, Bruna Cristina Dos Santos et al. "Evaluation of the efficacy of probiotic VSL#3 and synbiotic VSL#3 and yacon-based product in reducing oxidative stress and intestinal permeability in mice induced to colorectal carcinogenesis." *Journal of food science*, 10.1111/1750-3841.15690. 24 Mar. 2021, doi:10.1111/1750-3841.15690

large intestine. SFCAs benefit the health of the digestive tract and improve glucose homeostasis and insulin sensitivity. Also noteworthy, some prebiotic compounds have a near pharmaceutical-grade impact. Specifically, modified fruit pectin has potent anti-inflammatory effects and neutralizes galectin-3, a protein involved in inflammation and tissue fibrosis.

Synbiotics

Synbiotics refers to the combination of prebiotics and probiotics to enhance the viability of the live strains and their successful delivery to the gut microbiome—essentially a delivery strategy analogous to enteric-coated tablets. While the concept is relatively new, there is early scientific validation for its efficacy.[173]

Nutrition: Doctor-Patient Talking Points

Key goals for your nutritional strategy include
- Cultivating a nutrient-dense diet that supports your nutritional needs. This will be primarily plant-based, actively avoid processed carbohydrates and sugar, grain oils, and will de-emphasize animal sources, though periodic fish consumption can be a useful addition.
- If you already have a chronic illness or systemic inflammation (e.g., obesity), employing nutritional interventions can help moderate or reverse your symptoms. *Note: Useful supplement strategies will be covered in more detail later in the chapter.*
- Adopting nutritional strategies to enhance immune function, reduce illness duration and severity and promote healthy aging.
- Recognizing that stress, infection, trauma, chronic disease, and aging are all associated with reduced nutritional,

---

173 Hadi, Amir et al. "Efficacy of synbiotic interventions on blood pressure: a systematic review and meta-analysis of clinical trials." *Critical reviews in food science and nutrition*, 1-11. 22 Feb. 2021, doi:10.1080/10408398.2021.1888278

redox, and immune status. Intervening to address any diagnosed or projected nutritional deficit is an important adjunct to any medical intervention.

Reimagining the Doctor-Patient Relationship: A Conversation about Aging

The elderly are heavy consumers of healthcare services. An estimated 85% of adults over age 65 have one or more chronic diseases. Nine out of 10 report taking a prescription medicine, with over half taking four or more. Though controversial, some have called for aging to be classified as a disease, with the implication that it can be treated, managed, and perhaps even reversed. Common features of aging include

- Declining glutathione levels
- Declining NAD+ levels
- Reduced microbiome diversity
- Increased inflammation (inflammaging)
- Mitochondrial dysfunction
- Muscle loss (sarcopenia)
- Bone loss/reduced bone mineral density (osteopenia/osteoporosis)
- Frailty (weight loss, reduced strength, balance, gait, walking speed, etc.)
- Reduced immune function (immunosenescence)
- Reduced stress resilience
- Shortened cellular telomeres
- Cellular senescence
- Reduced DNA repair capacity
- Loss of function (hearing, eyesight, cognition)

While most of these issues are broadly accepted as inevitable, they are all linked to redox imbalance and oxidative stress. All have potential interventions that could delay their onset in service of healthier aging.

Aging: Doctor-Patient Talking Points

Few people reach old age without some limitations. Question: What are you obligated to accept, and what would you like to work on? Your answer will shape this conversation. Suggestions:
- Identify your big picture goals. Examples: "Live well" into old age and die at home. Minimize my use of prescription drugs.
- Cultivate an age-appropriate set of resilience practices as described in Chapter 7.
- Keep moving and exercising until the day you die, with increased emphasis on walking, strength training, balance, and flexibility exercises such as yoga.
- Monitor NLR and other inflammation biomarkers. Treat as necessary.
- Eat a nutrient-dense diet that includes plenty of resistant starch, soluble and insoluble fiber.
- Stay connected with friends and loved ones
- Stay intellectually engaged.
- Drink plenty of water
- Address sleep issues if you have them.
- Address disease-specific concerns in conversation with your doctor and nutritionist.
- Think about what it means to "die well." Develop plans and strategies to maximize the chances that you get to do it.

Note: There are some useful aging-related supplement strategies later in the chapter. An in-depth treatment of aging and redox imbalance is beyond the scope of this book. You can find more in-depth material on the redoxhealth.org website.

Reimagining the Doctor-Patient Relationship: A Conversation about Prescription Drugs, Over-the-Counter Meds, and Supplements

This conversation is perhaps the least likely to happen in a North American/Western medicine context, at least not in the way I would envision it. The twentieth century could rightly be characterized as the heyday of pharmaceutical medicine, when we explored both the promise and limitations of prescription medications. In the process, we created a powerful, lucrative industry with a vested interest in the continuation of the reigning medical paradigm, with its 55,000-plus diseases and protocols reliant on pills and procedures.

Despite some of the borderline miraculous achievements of the prior century (e.g., the virtual elimination of infectious disease as a major cause of mortality[174]), it is reasonable to observe that we learned to intervene with pharmaceuticals with a very limited understanding of how the body and disease actually works. Thus, we exited the twentieth century with epidemic obesity and diabetes and rising neurodegenerative, neuropsychiatric, and autoimmune disease rates. The US declines in heart disease, stroke rates,[175] [176] benefited substantially from dramatic declines in US smoking rates.

Furthermore, the idea that our pharmaceutical interventions are extending lifespan and healthspan is to say the least, controversial and comes at a great financial cost and with significant side effects. The current epidemic of prescription painkiller abuse has actually *reduced* US lifespan statistics for the first time in recent memory.

In the twenty-first century, scientists have made incredible strides in understanding how the body and its disease

---

[174] "Achievements in Public Health, 1900-1999: Control of Infectious Diseases." https://www.cdc.gov/mmwr/preview/mmwrhtml/mm4829a1.htm

[175] "Achievements in Public Health, 1900-1999: Decline in Deaths from Heart Disease and Stroke — United States, 1900-1999." https://www.cdc.gov/mmwr/preview/mmwrhtml/mm4830a1.htm

[176] Siegel, R.L., Miller, K.D. and Jemal, A. "Cancer statistics, 2020." CA A Cancer J Clin, 70: 7-30 (2020). doi.org/10.3322/caac.21590

processes work. Paradoxically, the more we learn, the clearer it becomes that chronic use and overuse of pharmaceutical and over-the-counter medicines are both problematic and largely unnecessary if appropriate diet, lifestyle, stress reduction/management, and nutritional interventions are taken. While I recognize that is a controversial statement—fighting words if you are invested in the pharmaceutical/medical paradigm—I can imagine living out my life with no or minimal use of prescription or even over-the-counter drugs.

Prescription Drugs

If you see your doctor regularly, odds are good that you are on multiple medications, especially as you age. In a redox imbalance treatment paradigm, we coordinate with our healthcare providers to minimize our dependence on prescription medication through diminished stress burden and enhanced stress resilience.

Using the ClinCalc "Top 200 Drugs of 2019" list, we can see what conditions drive prescription sales. The top 200 prescribed drugs generated 2.75 billion prescriptions in 2016 in the US alone. The top 100 prescription drugs generated over 2 billion of those 2.75 billion. Here's how the top 100 broke out by disease/condition:

Disease/Condition	Prescriptions
Hypertension	542,393,102
Cardiovascular disease / dyslipidemia	249,191,857
Diabetes	172,143,800
Pain	170,606,695
GERD	137,887,273
Seizure/bipolar/schizophrenia	114,557,335
Hypothyroidism	114,344,324
Allergies/antihistamines	85,701,343
Asthma/COPD	77,926,617
Antibiotics	63,779,524

ADHD	40,533,727
Anticoagulants	40,116,933
Enlarged prostate, BPH	32,833,515
Birth control	28,040,863
Muscle relaxants	25,245,375
Inflammation/steroids	23,242,849
Insomnia	19,102,809
Anemia	16,675,003
Gout, kidney stones	15,227,146
Hypoparathyroidism	14,608,444
Menopause/HRT	13,361,413
Osteoporosis	10,576,011
Glaucoma	9,879,869
Chemotherapy/anti-nausea	8,450,779
Dementia/Alzheimer's	7,761,701
Total Prescriptions:	**2,034,188,307**

I have two observations to share in light of this list. First, except for birth control, all of these prescriptions are designed to mitigate the symptoms of oxidative-stress-driven conditions. Thus, if we could help a broad swath of the population restore healthy redox status, many, if not most of these prescriptions would eventually become unnecessary.

Second, global pharmaceutical industry revenue has surpassed $1 trillion annually. About one-third of that revenue comes from the US, though the US represents barely 4 percent of the world's population and ranks forty-fifth[177] globally in life expectancy. Pharmaceutical disease management is costly, and it's not working very well. I don't expect a trillion-dollar industry to acknowledge that or change its behavior. By focusing on stress reduction, stress management, diet, nutrition, and lifestyle, doctors can minimize their patients' use and need for pharmaceuticals.

---

177 World Population Review, 2017 Data

Medications: Doctor-Patient Talking Points

- You can live a longer, healthier life while using fewer pharmaceuticals, but it requires that you adopt and maintain a healthy diet and lifestyle, with a robust collection of resilience habits as described in the previous chapter.
- Ideally, pharmaceuticals should be for acute health interventions. Unless you have a genetically-driven disease, or you've experienced some permanent damage (e.g., type 1 diabetes, gallbladder removal), be wary of the notion of "managing" disease with long-term prescription drugs unless you are unwilling or unable to address its root causes.
- Even in instances where pharmaceuticals are required, do not neglect the benefits of a healthy diet and lifestyle supported by a robust collection of resilience habits to overall health.
- Over-the-counter or non-prescription drugs are perceived as safe but can be dangerous if abused. Over-the-counter pain medications like ibuprofen, acetaminophen, and even aspirin are toxic stressors that damage the gut lining and lead to intestinal permeability. These drugs are called non-steroidal anti-inflammatory drugs (NSAIDs). As the acronym implies, we take these drugs to reduce inflammation and thereby pain.
- Safer alternatives include magnesium and peppermint oil (topical and/or aromatherapy) for headache and other pain,[178,179] and quercetin as a general anti-inflammatory.[180]

---

178 Göbel, H et al. "Oleum menthae piperitae (Pfefferminzöl) in der Akuttherapie des Kopfschmerzes vom Spannungstyp" [Peppermint oil in the acute treatment of tension-type headache]. *Schmerz (Berlin, Germany)* vol. 30,3 (2016): 295-310. doi:10.1007/s00482-016-0109-6

179 Akbari, Fatemeh et al. "Effect Of Peppermint Essence On The Pain And Anxiety Caused By Intravenous Catheterization In Cardiac Patients: A Randomized Controlled Trial." *Journal of pain research* vol. 12 2933-2939. 21 Oct. 2019, doi:10.2147/JPR.S226312

180 Valério, Daniel A et al. "Quercetin reduces inflammatory pain: inhibition of oxidative stress and cytokine production." *Journal of natural products* vol. 72,11 (2009): 1975-9. doi:10.1021/np900259y

Most polyphenols have anti-inflammatory, pain-reducing properties, with quercetin, curcumin, resveratrol, and kaempferol being the most studied. Finally, N-acetylcysteine has been shown to improve neuropathic pain via the inhibition of matrix metalloproteinases.[181]

Supplements and Nutraceuticals: Doctor-Patient Talking Points

- A person who is eating a nutrient-dense diet—mostly plants, minimally processed, low in inflammatory foods—can indeed meet most of their nutritional needs. These needs include vitamins, minerals, amino acids, phytonutrients (polyphenols, alkaloids, etc.), and macronutrients (fats/proteins/carbohydrates) from the food they eat. I think it's best to think of supplements as an intervention. If you don't need them, they don't help you and could be harmful. If they address a need, they can solve health issues or even save your life.
- That said, poor diet, sleep deficit, chronic stress, sedentary lifestyle, aging, and toxic and environmental stressors can damage and dysregulate your body to a place where intervention is necessary. While you should never assume you can solve all your problems with a pill, prescription, or supplement, knowing which supplements to take to address, specific issues can be incredibly useful.

Going Deeper: Useful Supplementation Strategies

Some readers might reasonably conclude that I am pro-supplement, but I would frame that differently. In my reading of a broad array of research, I have simply observed that much of what is needed to maintain and restore health homeostasis is available either through food or through non-prescription,

---

181 Li, Jiajie et al. "N-acetyl-cysteine attenuates neuropathic pain by suppressing matrix metalloproteinases." *Pain* vol. 157,8 (2016): 1711-23. doi:10.1097/j.pain.0000000000000575

non-patentable compounds: vitamins, minerals, amino acids, healthy fats, polyphenols, antimicrobials, and botanicals. That doesn't diminish the fact that there can be issues with supplements that consumers need to be aware of, such as lack of standardization and adulteration, particularly in herbal compounds. These concerns can largely be mitigated by purchasing from reputable manufacturers. A list of useful supplementation strategies include

NRF2 Stimulation

NRF2 is a gene pathway that upregulates cellular defenses and raises glutathione levels, making you more resilient to stress. Polyphenols like quercetin, rutin, resveratrol, pterostilbene, sulforaphane, EGCG, etc. are NRF2 stimulators. These are really interesting plant compounds that are useful for multiple issues because they are anti-inflammatory, anti-microbial, anti-cancer, antioxidant compounds with many other side benefits. They have these benefits largely because they stimulate NRF2.

AMPK activation

AMPK is a key regulator of metabolism, and recent studies have shown AMPK activation to precede NRF2 stimulation in compounds like berberine. Tandem stimulation of AMPK and NRF2 is a potent multi-target therapeutic strategy, addressing metabolic function and regulation, cellular defense and antioxidant capacity. Prominent AMPK activators include berberine, alpha-lipoic acid, metformin, quercetin, resveratrol, EGCG, and curcumin.

Glutathione Repletion

The glutathione pool (GSH/GSSG) needs to be maintained in a reduced state—high GSH, low GSSG. Under prolonged stress, glutathione levels can become depleted to the point that damage and dysregulation occur. Supplementing with glutathione precursors such as N-acetylcysteine, glycine, L-glutamine, and cofactors vitamin D3, B12, magnesium, zinc, selenium, and alpha-lipoic acid, or with liposomal glutathione—all are useful glutathione repletion strategies that complement NRF2 stimulation.

NAD+ Repletion

NAD+ is a coenzyme responsible for regulating energy production in the mitochondria and facilitating sirtuin production. NAD+ levels are depleted by oxidative stress-driven DNA damage, overconsumption of processed carbs and sugars, aging, and/or overconsumption of antioxidants. NAD+ (and glutathione) levels are known to fall with age. However, you can restore NAD+ levels by supplementing with nicotinamide riboside or nicotinamide mononucleotide, variants of niacin/vitamin B3.

Addressing Nutritional Deficits

There's good evidence that much of the country has a subclinical magnesium deficiency and that it drives a wide range of health issues from heart disease to osteoarthritis. Nutritional deficits can arise from stress, illness, prescription and nonprescription drug use, poor diet, and gut dysbiosis—imbalances in your intestinal bacteria. Malnutrition routinely accompanies critical illness, so it is reasonable to assume that the stresses that lead to critical illness also drive declining nutritional status, that malnutrition participates in the severity of the illness, and that addressing the malnutrition would be integral to the healing process.

Addressing Specific Ailments

Knowing that rutin helps with hemorrhoids and raises energy levels, or that quercetin is a natural antihistamine, or that taurine helps prevent age-related muscle loss, or that apple cider vinegar kills bacteria in the stomach and upper GI that cause acid reflux and heartburn is useful information. There are literally thousands of these strategies that have reasonable scientific evidence for their efficacy. Always check PubMed.gov before trying something, always start slowly to avoid nasty surprises, and never assume that more would be better. I've found many strategies that work for me and my issues. Your mileage may vary.

Immune Boosting

In the last chapter, under "Preparing for illness and infection," I mentioned curating a collection of antimicrobial compounds and immunonutrients to fight colds and upper respiratory infections. The same nutrients/minerals/amino acids that help you maintain healthy antioxidant capacity/glutathione levels also help you keep your immune system tuned and effective. These compounds include magnesium, zinc, vitamin D3, vitamin B12, taurine, arginine, N-acetylcysteine, etc. Also, there are useful antimicrobial compounds that kill not just bacteria but also viruses and fungi. These include oil of oregano, garlic extract, olive leaf extract, black seed oil, elderberry, Umcka, bee propolis, lactoferrin, and many more. I use these when I feel a cold or respiratory infection coming on and stopping or shortening the duration and/or severity. Anecdotally, they work well, and there is a reasonable body of research evidence for their efficacy, which I have used to choose the most effective compounds.

Anti-Aging

In the prior chapter, I also alluded to curating a collection of anti-aging strategies. In general terms, our resilience habits = our anti-aging strategy, but several supplement strategies are getting attention in the field of anti-aging that we can touch on based on broad categories. Some supplements may appear more than once because they are pleiotropic/multi-target compounds:

NFR2 activators

The decline of NRF2 expression is a key driver of aging, allowing increased ROS accumulation in cells, with resulting redox imbalance that increases DNA damage, senescence, and other cellular pathologies of aging, and raises the risk of cancer, neurodegeneration, and other aging-related diseases.

Compounds and activities that activate NRF2, including the majority of our proposed resilience habits, are viewed as anti-aging. Supplements that activate NRF2 include
- Quercetin
- Resveratrol
- Rutin
- Sulforaphane
- EGCG
- Pterostilbene
- Curcumin
- Berberine
- And many, many more...

Some researchers have voiced concern that activation of NRF2 can protect cancer cells from immune-targeted destruction, and indeed, the adaptive benefits of NRF2 occur at low levels of stimulation. That said, the natural NRF2 activators are almost universally viewed as anti-cancer compounds, inducing senescence in cancer cells, killing cancer stem cells, inhibiting telomerase activity, and/or acting radiosensitizers and chemosensitizers alongside conventional therapies.

Glutathione repletion and other redox related nutritional interventions

While I have generally preferred NRF2 stimulation as a means of raising intracellular glutathione levels, a recent study involving older adults showed that supplementing with a combination of glycine and N-acetylcysteine (both rate-limiting precursors of glutathione) over 24 weeks corrected a deficit of GSH in red blood cells and improved:
- Oxidative stress and mitochondrial dysfunction
- Inflammation
- Endothelial dysfunction
- Insulin- resistance
- Genomic- damage
- Cognition
- Strength
- Gait- speed

- Exercise capacity
- Body- fat mass and waist- circumference

Benefits declined after stopping the supplementation for 12 weeks.[182] The study's significance is not that these two amino acids are somehow a silver bullet for aging. Rather, it signifies that older adults are prone to glutathione deficiencies that, if addressed, mitigate a broad range of age-related pathologies. That's a big deal, both as a specific therapy and as a general principle that addressing nutritional deficits can mitigate aging symptoms. Many of these symptoms are both common and distressing, significantly affecting quality of life and the ability to function independently. We know that there are many other common nutritional deficits associated with aging, including taurine,[183] zinc,[184] selenium,[185] magnesium,[186] vitamin B12, folate,[187] vitamin D,[188] vitamin K.[189] This is a

---

182 Kumar, Premranjan et al. "Glycine and N-acetylcysteine (GlyNAC) supplementation in older adults improves glutathione deficiency, oxidative stress, mitochondrial dysfunction, inflammation, insulin resistance, endothelial dysfunction, genotoxicity, muscle strength, and cognition: Results of a pilot clinical trial." *Clinical and translational medicine* vol. 11,3 (2021): e372. doi:10.1002/ctm2.372

183 Chupel, Matheus Uba et al. "Taurine supplementation reduces myeloperoxidase and matrix-metalloproteinase-9 levels and improves the effects of exercise in cognition and physical fitness in older women." Amino acids vol. 53,3 (2021): 333-345. doi:10.1007/s00726-021-02952-6

184 Wong, Carmen P et al. "Effects of zinc status on age-related T cell dysfunction and chronic inflammation." *Biometals : an international journal on the role of metal ions in biology, biochemistry, and medicine* vol. 34,2 (2021): 291-301. doi:10.1007/s10534-020-00279-5

185 Rita Cardoso, Bárbara et al. "Selenium status in elderly: relation to cognitive decline." *Journal of trace elements in medicine and biology : organ of the Society for Minerals and Trace Elements (GMS)* vol. 28,4 (2014): 422-6. doi:10.1016/j.jtemb.2014.08.009

186 Dominguez, Ligia J et al. "Magnesium in Infectious Diseases in Older People." *Nutrients Vol.* 13,1 180. 8 Jan. 2021, doi:10.3390/nu13010180

187 Matthews, J H. "Cobalamin and folate deficiency in the elderly." *Bailliere's clinical haematology* vol. 8,3 (1995): 679-97. doi:10.1016/s0950-3536(05)80226-4

188 D'Amelio P. "Vitamin D Deficiency and Risk of Metabolic Syndrome in Aging Men." World J Mens Health. 2021 Apr;39(2):291-301. doi: 10.5534/wjmh.200189. Epub 2021 Jan 26. PMID: 33663024; PMCID: PMC7994656.

189 Dal Canto, Elisa et al. "The Association of Vitamin D and Vitamin K Status with Subclinical Measures of Cardiovascular Health and All-Cause Mortality in Older Adults: The Hoorn Study." *The Journal of nutrition* vol. 150,12 (2020): 3171-3179. doi:10.1093/jn/nxaa293

partial list. Nonetheless, the idea that addressing multiple diagnosed nutritional deficiencies could significantly enhance quality of life in aging is potentially game-changing.

Senolytics

Senolytics, compounds that destroy or remove senescent cells (aging cells that no longer divide), have attracted significant attention in the anti-aging research community. Most recently, trials using Quercetin and Dasatinib, a senolytic drug, showed symptom relief in pulmonary fibrosis and a reduction of senescent cells in the adipose tissue of patients with diabetic kidney disease.[190] The attraction of this approach is that senescent cells secrete pro-inflammatory compounds that damage and distress surrounding cells. Thus, removing them can alleviate certain disease symptoms and potentially slow the progression of the disease. This phenomenon, known as senescence-associated secretory phenotype (SASP), plays a role in its pathology. Natural senolytic compounds include

- Polyphenols
  - Curcumin
  - EGCG
  - Fisetin
  - Genisteine
  - Phloretin
  - Pterostilbene
  - Quercetin
  - Resveratrol
- Alkaloids
  - Berberine
  - Piperlongumine
- Terpenoids

---

190 Hickson, LaTonya J et al. "Senolytics decrease senescent cells in humans: Preliminary report from a clinical trial of Dasatinib plus Quercetin in individuals with diabetic kidney disease." *EBioMedicine* vol. 47 (2019): 446-456. doi:10.1016/j.ebiom.2019.08.069

Telomerase Activators

Shortened cellular telomeres are a feature of aging and senescence in cells. Upregulating telomerase has been proposed as a possible therapeutic for lengthening telomeres and contributing to slowing or reversing aging. Research has identified several telomerase activators, but to date, there have been no clinical trials that confirm efficacy in humans.

- *Centella asiatica* (CA), a 2019 study, showed CA raised telomerase levels nearly ninefold. Commonly known as gotu kola, centella asiatica has a long history of medical use in Ayurveda and Chinese traditional medicine.
- Oleanolic acid (OA), in the same study, OA came in second, raising telomerase nearly sixfold.[191]

Also significant, telomerase inhibitors are viewed as anti-cancer therapeutics. Telomerase is hijacked by cancer cells as a mechanism to ensure ongoing cell division. Notably, curcumin inhibits telomerase in cancer cells.

NAD+ repletion. NAD+ is part of the NAD+/NADH redox couple. Functionally, NAD+ is a key oxidant regulator of metabolism and raw material for sirtuin production and the DNA repair enzyme poly(ADP-ribose) polymerase (PARP). NAD+ and NAD+-dependent enzyme levels fall with age, contributing to mitochondrial dysfunction, genomic instability, and numerous diseases associated with metabolism and oxidative stress, including cancer, diabetes, and sarcopenia. Key strategies for NAD+ repletion include supplementing with precursors nicotinamide riboside and nicotinamide mononucleotide. Though lower profile (and way cheaper!), taurine supplementation has also been shown to increase the NAD+/NADH ratio while taurine deficiency, common in old age, raises it. This at least raises the prospect that falling NAD+ levels in aging are partially the result of taurine depletion. Other contributors would include oxidative

---

191 Tsoukalas, Dimitris et al. "Discovery of potent telomerase activators: Unfolding new therapeutic and anti-aging perspectives." *Molecular medicine reports* vol. 20,4 (2019): 3701-3708. doi:10.3892/mmr.2019.10614

stress-driven DNA damage and associated upregulation of PARP and overconsumption/production of glucose, and the activation of the Polyol Pathway.

Sirtuin upregulation

Sirtuins are a family of NAD+-dependent enzymes that play key roles in cellular defense, including DNA repair, regulation of mitochondrial biogenesis and function, antioxidant protection via upregulation of antioxidant enzymes superoxide dismutase (SOD), catalase and glutathione peroxidase, and metabolism of glucose and lipids.[192] Sirtuins are also involved in various resilience pathways described in chapter 7, including AMPK, NRF2, PGC1a, and FOXO. Natural sirtuin activators include
- Fisetin
- Quercetin
- Curcumin
- Berberine
- Resveratrol

Autophagy/mitophagy regulation

Autophagy, literally "self-eating," is a cellular recycling process that promotes cellular homeostasis and quality control by removing waste, excess or misfolded proteins, and damaged organelles. Mitophagy describes an analogous process in your mitochondria. Dysregulation of autophagy/mitophagy is increasingly viewed as a pathological mechanism in multiple diseases, including cardiovascular and lung diseases, Alzheimer's, Parkinson's, ALS, Huntington's, multiple sclerosis, and other neurological diseases. Autophagy/mitophagy is broadly protective—a part of the cellular stress response, but when downregulated or insufficient under overwhelming stress, plays a role in cell death (apoptosis/necrosis) and, in the brain, neuroinflammation, neurodegeneration, and neuronal death. We see this in the

---

[192] Iside, Concetta, et al. "SIRT1 Activation by Natural Phytochemicals: An Overview." Frontiers in Pharmacology, vol. 11 (2020). doi:10.3389/fphar.2020.01225

diabetes-associated cognitive decline. Diabetes-induced high glucose in the brain activates autophagy as an acute protective response, but one ultimately insufficient to prevent neuronal death from prolonged hyperglycemia.[193] Polyphenols again emerge as ideal regulators of autophagy/mitophagy in that they positively regulate redox status (via NRF2) and mitochondrial function (via AMPK) while activating autophagy. Polyphenols with known roles in autophagy regulation include

- Apigenin
- Curcumin
- EGCG
- Quercetin
- Resveratrol
- Rutin

It's notable that, as with senescence, many of these compounds can situationally inhibit or promote autophagy, which is potentially useful in cancer prevention and treatment.

Fitness

Exercise physiology, which is particularly interested in optimizing physical performance and training efficacy, has shown that maintaining healthy antioxidant status is useful for exercise recovery, so you may find some benefits from NRF2 stimulation. Also, amino acid supplementation (branched-chain amino acids, taurine, creatine, glycine, etc.) may fall into the category of addressing nutritional deficits for someone who is working out heavily or lifting weights.

Reimagining the Doctor-Patient Relationship: A Conversation about Genetics, Epigenetics, and Signaling

While the ability to sequence the human genome hasn't immediately ushered in the age of personalized medicine, progress is being made, both in understanding what genetic

---

[193] Wu, Yanqing et al. "Autophagy Activation is Associated with Neuroprotection in Diabetes-associated Cognitive Decline." *Aging and disease* vol. 10,6 1233-1245. 1 Dec. 2019, doi:10.14336/AD.2018.1024

variations are associated with specific ailments and how various treatment strategies might work differently for each individual. Consumer genetic testing from companies like 23andMe and ancestry.com is cheap by medical standards, under $100 in many cases, but covers only the most common single nucleotide pairs (SNPs).

More robust "whole genome" tests have dropped into the $300 range and will cover every genetic variant in your genome. At the time of publication, Nebula Genomics offered such a test, with a strong privacy policy and blockchain security. Adding a lifetime subscription to their analysis services platform costs an extra $700, but considering such testing cost several thousand dollars without analysis, this is a pretty amazing bargain. I've ordered it on an introductory promotion. I will update this section when I have a more informed opinion. Still, the initial takeaway is that though immature, the era of whole-genome testing for medical purposes has arrived.

Genetics: Doctor-Patient Talking Points

While genetics would be viewed as a medical specialty in the current paradigm, your primary care physician and health system will likely be asking you to get a full DNA sequence thanks to falling prices and the increasing value of having such information. I would envision the doctor-patient conversation including some of the following talking points:

- Based on your whole genome test and analysis, we will discuss any relevant health-related issues flagged in the report.
- You will typically find a lot of conflicting information in your genetic profile—some genes that might make you more likely to get a disease, such as Alzheimer's, and others that are protective.
- Researchers have identified "common risk alleles" through genome-wide association studies. Examples include
    ◦ Factor V Leiden, a risk for deep venous thrombosis, occurs in 3 to 8 percent of people of European descent.

- MTHFR polymorphisms occur in 60 to 70 percent of the general population
- Studies of genetic mutations of the MTHFR (methylenetetrahydrofolate reductase) gene, which is involved in DNA synthesis and methylation, have proven fruitful. People with MTHFR mutations have trouble metabolizing B vitamins and need to take them in their methyl forms (e.g., methylfolate/B9, methylcobalamin/B12). For example, the MTHFR C677T polymorphism is associated with elevated blood homocysteine levels. Accompanying inflammation is involved in migraine, birth defects, and adverse pregnancy outcomes. Taking methyl forms of B9 and B12 reduces homocysteine levels.
- Variations of the CYP2D6 allele can cause certain people to be "rapid metabolizers" or "ultra-rapid metabolizers" of certain drugs, making them either dangerous or ineffective.
- Genetic polymorphisms will vary by ethnicity, which can mean that disease prevalence or the efficacies of certain therapies will also vary by ethnicity.
- You can explore more about genetic involvement in a condition you or a loved one might have by going to PubMed.org and searching for "polymorphism <your disease>" or "risk allele <your disease>."
- Genetics is not destiny. How you live is equally important because of the environmental/experiential impact on gene expression through epigenetic modulation.

Caveat: This area is evolving rapidly, so do your research and don't assume I've given you anything more than a teaser.

Epigenetics: Doctor-Patient Talking Points

To use an analogy, if the genome is hardware, the epigenome is software. It controls how genes are expressed. Our earlier discussions of resilience habits are entirely based on the notion that activation of key genetic pathways changes the epigenetic

state of a wide range of resilience-related genes. Your doctor will want you to know the following:
- What used to be scientific heresy is now scientific fact: epigenetic changes in our cells are happening all the time to maintain homeostasis while allowing us to constantly adapt to our changing environment.
- In oxidative eustress (good stress), low-level oxidative stressors initiate an adaptive response that upregulates gene pathways such as NRF2, AMPK, FOXO, PGC1a, and HO-1 and makes you more stress-resilient.
- In a state of redox imbalance, the opportunities to switch on pathological genes are increased.
- Genetics is not destiny. Epigenetic changes are not necessarily permanent.
- At the same time, genetics matter, and epigenetic changes can be passed on to the next generation.

Going Deeper: Epigenetics, Signaling, Therapeutic Pathways, and Transcription Factors

A motivated patient may want to know more about the underlying mechanisms involved in regulating and dysregulating their bodily systems. The concept of pathways is a relatively new but foundational area in systems biology. For our purposes, a pathway is a sequence of actions among molecules in a cell that lead to a particular outcome or change in the cell. A transcription factor (TF) is a regulatory protein whose role is to control a gene target's transcription from DNA to messenger RNA. Wikipedia explains it well:

> "The function of TFs is to regulate—turn on and off—genes in order to make sure that they are expressed in the right cell at the right time and in the right amount throughout the life of the cell and the organism."[194]

---

194 Wikipedia contributors. "Transcription factor." *Wikipedia, The Free Encyclopedia*. Wikipedia, The Free Encyclopedia, 11 Sep. 2020. Web. 14 Oct. 2020.

Research into these biochemical pathways over the past two decades has provided windows into disease initiation and progression. This area is new enough that many of the best strategies for manipulating these pathways are plant-based compounds such as curcumin, berberine, quercetin, and resveratrol. While there is also an increasing number of pharmaceutical options for manipulating gene pathways, they are not necessarily preferred over the natural compounds, which often have long histories of therapeutic use, a broad array of health benefits, good safety profiles, and few side effects.

Pathway	Description	Benefits	Risks
NRF2-ARE	Regulates stress resilience	Stimulation upregulates cellular defenses, preventing damage and dysregulation	Concerns about making cancer cells more resilient
AMPK	Regulates metabolism, mitochondrial function	Stimulation improves mitochondrial biogenesis, reduces mitochondrial ROS	
NF-κB	Activates the immune system	Plays important roles in cell regulation—DNA transcription, cytokine production, cell survival	Dysregulated NF-κB can play a role in inflammatory diseases and cancer.

JNK	Controls cellular response to harmful stimuli, frequently leading to cell death (apoptosis)	Programmed cell death is an important function in the health homeostasis of a multicellular organism.	JNK signaling is involved in some cancers and neurodegenerative diseases.
MAPK/ERK	Plays roles in cellular proliferation and differentiation.	Cell differentiation is an important process to health and healthy aging.	Dysregulated MAPK/ERK signaling can lead to cancer and plays a role in Alzheimer's and Parkinson's disease.
P38 aka P38 MAPK	Plays a major regulatory role in endothelial cell oxidative stress response, including effects on vascular tone, permeability, DNA damage response, apoptosis, and senescence.	Healthy P38 signaling plays a central role in maintaining cardiovascular in response to stressors.	Dysregulated P38 plays a role in cancer initiation and progression through upregulation of inflammatory mediators and atherosclerosis.
mTOR	Mammalian target of rapamycin is a central regulator of mammalian metabolism and physiology. It is dysregulated in obesity, diabetes, depression, and autoimmunity.	Inhibition of mTOR is associated with life extension.	mTOR is frequently upregulated in autoimmune diseases such as lupus.

Polyol	Plays a role in glucose metabolism.	Overconsumption of glucose could be toxic, and the polyol pathway provides a mechanism for dealing with excess glucose.	Overuse of the polyol pathway leads to excess oxidative stress, depletion of NAD+, and mitochondrial dysfunction.
Kynurenine	Plays a role in tryptophan metabolism.	Provides a secondary mechanism for raising NAD+ levels.	Overactivation causes neural oxidative stress and lower serotonin production and is associated with numerous mental health conditions and neurodegenerative diseases.
HIF1α	Hypoxia Inducible Factor 1a	Regulates the body's response to low oxygen situations—hypoxia.	Over-expression of HIF-1a is thought to play a role in cancer initiation and metastasis.
FOXO	Forkhead box proteins	FOXO proteins are significant players in aging and longevity	Silencing of certain FOXO genes (e.g., FOXO3a) can lead to carcinogenesis.
HO-1	Heme Oxygenase-1	HO-1 controls the degradation of heme. Upregulation of HO-1 is generally associated with positive health outcomes, reducing oxidative stress.	HO activity is low in obesity. Upregulating HO-1 increases bilirubin production, which has antioxidant properties but is high in neonatal jaundice.

Reimagining the Doctor-Patient Relationship: A Conversation about Symptoms and Pathologies

In patient forums across the globe, the following post or some variation occurs with depressing frequency: "In recent months, I've been experiencing symptoms X, Y, and Z. My doctors haven't been able to give me a diagnosis, and it seems like the symptoms are getting worse. I'm really frustrated. Any ideas?"

The doctors may indeed be unable to give a definitive diagnosis, but that is actually the fault of the Western medical disease model, which treats diseases as though they were objectively real and distinct, rather than labels we put on the symptoms arising from multiple intersecting stressors and pathologies.

Core Pathologies: Redox Imbalance and Downstream Damage/Dysregulation

The idea that redox imbalance is an insufficient but necessary cause in disease pathology has a corollary: In my surveying of the most recent decades of research, I've identified the following core pathologies (shared earlier), each with pathological associations stemming from oxidative stress/ redox imbalance:

- Cellular pathologies including
  - Mitochondrial damage/dysfunction
  - Endoplasmic reticulum stress/proteome dysregulation
  - DNA Damage in the nucleus or mitochondria
  - Calcium loading/calcium channel dysregulation
  - Insulin resistance/glucose intolerance
  - Leptin resistance
  - Cell life cycle dysregulation affecting:
    - Apoptosis
    - Angiogenesis
    - Mutagenesis
    - Necrosis

- Replication
- Senescence
- Autophagy
- Tissue pathologies
  - Fibrosis
  - Sclerosis
  - Tissue remodeling
  - Vascular permeability/endothelial dysfunction
  - Cellular adhesion
  - Edema
  - Tumorigenesis
- Systemic dysregulation
  - Chronic HPA axis activation/dysregulation
  - Chronic sympathetic nervous system activation/sympathetic–parasympathetic imbalance
  - Chronic renin-angiotensin-aldosterone–system activation/dysregulation
  - Chronic immune system activation/dysregulation
  - Haematological system dysregulation
    - Hemolysis
    - Clotting/thrombosis
    - Anti-coagulation
    - Anemia
  - Intestinal permeability, gut barrier dysfunction
  - Dysbiosis
  - Musculoskeletal system dysregulation
    - Bone resorption/loss/remodeling
    - Muscle loss/weakness
  - Low/dysregulated nutritional status
  - Toxic load/loss of detoxification capacity
  - Genetic/epigenetic stress and signaling dysregulation
  - Obesity/metabolic dysregulation

In the majority of these pathologies, a normal physiological function is simply dysregulated in a manner that makes it pathological. In a redox treatment paradigm, I propose that most chronic diseases are just symptoms of underlying pathologies that result in clinical symptoms. Thus, hypertension is a symptom of:

- Cellular redox imbalance leading to mitochondrial dysfunction, endoplasmic reticulum stress, and pathological signaling (e.g., NF-κB activation, P38/MAPK activation).
- Chronic HPA axis activation/dysregulation leading to elevated serum catecholamine levels and:
- Chronic sympathetic nervous system activation/sympathetic-parasympathetic imbalance leading to vasoconstriction from:
- Chronic renin-angiotensin-aldosterone-system activation/dysregulation leading to hyperaldosteronism, dysregulation of electrolytes (e.g., magnesium, calcium, phosphorus, potassium, sodium), and elevated renin and angiotensin II levels.
- Chronic immune system activation/dysregulation and elevated oxidative stress leading to:
    - Intestinal permeability and gut dysbiosis leading to systemic inflammation.[195]
    - Vascular permeability/endothelial dysfunction, leading to fluid retention, arterial stiffness, low NO availability, and atherosclerosis.
    - Low/dysregulated nutritional status—low magnesium, low taurine, likely dysregulated sodium-potassium balance.
- Genetic/epigenetic stress and signaling dysregulation leading to downregulation of endothelial eNOS levels and alterations of blood pressure-associated miRNA levels.[196]

Hypertension responds very well to a whole-food, plant-

---

195 Santisteban, Monica M et al. "Hypertension-Linked Pathophysiological Alterations in the Gut." *Circulation research* vol. 120,2 (2017): 312-323. doi:10.1161/CIRCRESAHA.116.309006

196 Kontaraki, Joanna E et al. "MicroRNA-9 and microRNA-126 expression levels in patients with essential hypertension: potential markers of target-organ damage." *Journal of the American Society of Hypertension : JASH* vol. 8,6 (2014): 368-75. doi:10.1016/j.jash.2014.03.324

based, nutrient-dense diet[197] in large part because such diets address all of the above pathologies by reducing dietary stressors and enhancing nutritional status and antioxidant capacity via NRF2-stimulating phytonutrients. It's also useful to understand how to intervene via nutritional supplementation to modulate these underlying pathologies because they are root cause issues in hypertension and thousands of other diseases.

Other Disease-Specific Discussions

While tackling the treatment strategies for the 155,000+ individual diseases is beyond the scope of this book, the list of underlying disease pathologies in the section above is much more manageable and provides a starting place for any exploration of disease.

For those with an insatiable desire to learn more, I will post material deemed too in-depth for a consumer book on my website: https://redoxhealth.org.

Treating Redox Imbalance: Summing Up

Given that we do not currently treat redox imbalance, this chapter has largely been an exercise in envisioning a future where we did treat redox imbalance. Key takeaways from that exercise include
- We already have a large body of knowledge about how to modulate redox status.
- Since redox imbalance is an insufficient but necessary cause, treating it has significant potential for improving overall health outcomes.
- There will necessarily be other accompanying causes,

---

197 Alexander, Sarah et al. "A plant-based diet and hypertension." *Journal of geriatric cardiology : JGC* vol. 14,5 (2017): 327-330. doi:10.11909/j.issn.1671-5411.2017.05.014

such as nutritional deficits, mitochondrial dysfunction, proteome dysregulation, immune system dysregulation, and other systemic dysregulation. Those accompanying causes will also have linkages to oxidative stress.
- Oxidative stress plays a key role in a broad range of pathological processes including pain, inflammation, fibrosis, sclerosis, rash, cellular adhesion, senescence, necrosis, apoptosis, DNA damage, telomere shortening, tumorigenesis, mutagenesis, dysbiosis, endothelial hyperpermeability, gut hyperpermeability, and bone and muscle loss. Most of these increase in prevalence with aging along with rising oxidative stress levels.
- Our doctors will have a greater interest in both the underlying stressors contributing to our health issues and the elimination, mitigation, and management of those stressors. The concept of the Exposome and its impact on epigenetics and our genome expression will enter the doctor-patient conversation.
- Relatively new oxidative stress-relevant biomarkers such as NLR, SII, and something analogous to the Allostatic Load Index, will serve as early warnings of redox imbalance and allow us to intervene earlier, thereby preventing comorbid diseases before they happen.
- Consumers' ability to gather clinically relevant health data and monitor health status in real-time is expanding rapidly. This needs to be leveraged to improve health outcomes.
- Our doctors will emphasize maintaining and bolstering stress resilience to enhance our current health status while making us more resistant to future disease and health crises.
- Nutrition will play a much larger role in health maintenance and management than it currently does. Furthermore, the interdependent nature of redox status, nutritional status, and immune status will be increasingly acknowledged and leveraged therapeutically.
- While secondary to nutrient-dense eating, nutritional supplementation will play an important role as an

intervention to address nutritional deficits and bolster immune and redox status, particularly in acute conditions and aging.
- Full genome signaling will become routine and begin to inform therapeutics, often employing epigenetic strategies to manipulate gene-regulating pathways such as AMPK, NRF2, and FOXO.
- Our increasing ability to effectively manage and treat redox imbalance and its downstream effects will significantly improve healthspan and quality of life in aging.

Perhaps ironically, many of these changes will happen regardless of whether there is an explicit acknowledgment of redox imbalance as a root cause of disease simply because accumulating scientific evidence is pushing the industry in these directions. That said, I believe the pace of progress and the health benefits that accrue will be greater when we finally do measure, diagnose, and treat redox imbalance.

Chapter 9

Moving Forward, Claiming the Benefits

It's hard to imagine a paradigm more entrenched than the western medical paradigm. So what do we do if, as an accumulating body of evidence indicates, redox imbalance really is the root cause of chronic disease and if redox signaling and the body's stress adaptation systems held the key to preventing and even curing disease? What if the tools and strategies from applying this information were free or low-cost and largely didn't involve prescription medications or surgery? And what if the reigning paradigm was resistant to this new information?

While I believe the evidence is compelling that redox imbalance should be at the center of the disease model and how we think about health and disease, I am also cognizant that there is much work to do before this becomes the dominant health paradigm. The purpose of this book is to help point "those with eyes to see" in the right direction. As with any journey, if you walk in the right direction, you will encounter and solve the right problems before you reach your destination. I am making the case through this book that recent scientific developments are showing us the right direction. The question remains, even if you're convinced, how do you act on that knowledge and claim the benefits?

Living Out Redox Health Principles on a Personal Level

In the near term, as I mentioned in chapter 8, the medical practitioners most philosophically amenable to redox health principles are in the field of functional medicine because of their commitment to a systems approach to health and interest in root causes. If I had ready access to a functional medicine doctor in my region, that's where I'd be going. I could see this being a very fruitful doctor-patient collaboration.

Beyond the doctor-patient relationship's basics, I have committed myself to live into and living out the principles I am espousing, albeit imperfectly, which I have framed as the redox health paradigm. Everyone will have their own take on what this might look like, but for me, it includes

- Minimizing my use of the healthcare system.
- Minimizing my use of pharmaceuticals.
- Cultivating a robust set of resilience habits including
  - Eating a nutrient-dense diet.
  - Exercising regularly.
  - Managing stress effectively.
  - Maintaining stress resilience by bolstering antioxidant capacity, nutritional status, and immune status.
- Thinking about life's challenges in terms of stress and their oxidative stress impact.
- Developing strategies to self-treat common maladies, including aging.
- Taking full advantage of technological advances in mobile health and continuous monitoring of an ever-broader array of biomarkers.
- Continuing to learn about how the body works, including my genetic and microbiome information.
- Moving intentionally and incrementally in the direction of pro-health decisions. This includes avoiding health-destroying activities.
- Dying well, preferably at home.

I realize that this is a difficult balancing act and that there are risks in taking this path, given that it is less mature. I accept those risks because I have already seen the benefits. Those benefits for me include

- Fewer respiratory infections.
- Fewer, shorter colds.
- Improved allergy control.
- Minimal health impacts from a type 2 diabetes diagnosis ten years ago—namely, no discernible vision or neuropathy impacts.
- Lower costs
- General good health despite a high-stress profession.

One of the most important benefits for me has been the sense of empowerment I feel from knowing more about what causes disease, how it progresses, having strategies to prevent and combat the most common health challenges, and the ability to research and learn about new ones.

In my experience, one of the most pernicious flaws of the current medical paradigm is the profound sense of disempowerment patients seeking help can experience. Whether it is waiting for weeks or months to see a specialist, months or even years for a diagnosis, waiting for relief from chronic pain, being told your condition has no known cause or cure, being diagnosed with multiple diseases, each with its own treatment protocol, or knowing that your treatment protocol has short-term side effects and/or dangerous long-term health impacts—any of these can leave the patient feeling helpless and powerless. I recognize that places like Cleveland Clinic and other research hospital systems are much more effective in many of these areas, but often at a high cost that cannot scale to a global population.

The knowledge that stress and oxidative stress cause disease is simple enough that most health consumers can grasp it. The knowledge that stress can be mitigated and managed, that redox imbalance can be modulated, those nutritional deficits can be predicted, measured, and addressed, that disease loops and pathologies can be identified and disrupted—these are profoundly empowering concepts. The patient can have vastly more agency and control over their health than in the current health paradigm. While that knowledge and empowerment also bring increased accountability, that's an exchange I would welcome.

A lower-cost healthcare paradigm has ramifications for health insurance and how we pay for care. Here again, patient empowerment and accountability are core values. Just as I want to minimize my use of the healthcare system, I want to minimize my contact with the health insurance system, with its bewildering complexity and high cost. Though I consider myself fairly liberal politically, given the opportunity, I would choose a health savings account (HSA) with catastrophic insurance as my preferred insurance model. This approach makes me accountable for my health decisions and gives me greater control over my care choices. Assuming the redox-centric approach yields lower-cost healthcare, I benefit financially.

One of the challenges under the current healthcare paradigm is that standard insurance policies do not generally cover nutritional and redox therapies. While the therapies I use are generally quite inexpensive, I recognize that many people struggle to pay for health insurance and have limited funds to put toward anything beyond the premiums.

Thinking Bigger

At a personal level, redox imbalance as a root cause of chronic disease and the associated redox health paradigm points us towards strategies that should result in better mental and physical health at every stage of life for each of us individually and potentially for our families and friends. But I am also keenly aware of the broader implications, and they are vast. I plan to dive deeper into this topic in a later book, but as an exercise, ask yourself the following questions:

1. What does the fast-food industry look like when you accept that highly-processed, low-nutrient, preservative-laden foods and high-heat cooking (i.e., stuff fried in soybean oil) are major contributors to dietary oxidative stress?

2. What do ag and farm policies look like when you consider that processed grains, grain oil, grain-fed beef, and dairy are significant sources of dietary oxidative stress contributing to chronic inflammatory diseases, not to mention their environmental impact?

3. What does the pharmaceutical industry look like if people understand that most chronic diseases can be addressed by lifestyle changes, nutritional interventions, and unpatented natural compounds?

4. What does the food industry look like when there is broad recognition that their products, including soft drinks, grain oils, food additives, high fructose corn syrup and other added sugars, refined flour, are primary drivers of dietary oxidative stress and chronic disease?

5. How should labor policy change when there is broad understanding that long hours, lack of adequate vacation, shift work, and high-stress work environments are significant contributors to stress-driven chronic disease?

6. How should environmental policy change to acknowledge the key role of particulate matter air pollution and water pollution from industrial, agricultural, medical, and residential sources as health stressors?

7. How would large corporations' HR policy, benefits, wellness strategies change if they knew they could lower their healthcare costs by helping employees maintain a healthy redox status?

8. How would the medical industry change if we only spent 10% of GDP on healthcare instead of 20%, yet got better results?

9. How should the tech industry protect children and adult consumers from the stressors that technology has introduced into our lives, from excess screen time to work encroachments on non-work time to social media?

10. How would governmental policy in general change if leadership viewed the citizenry's health as a national security issue and an issue of economic competitiveness?

While I can't promise specific results, I think the science supports the possibility of better health outcomes at lower cost by following a redox health paradigm's principles. Getting there would have the potential for pretty dramatic impacts on some very large industries that contribute to and benefit from the unhealth of the global population. At the same time, there are also many instances of governments, industries, and entire economies that are threatened by rising healthcare costs and the declining mental and physical health status of employees and citizens.

While an in-depth discussion of all these issues is beyond this book's scope, I believe that it's important to think bigger. An individual can only do so much to improve their health. There are important roles for government, industry, religion, and non-governmental organizations in promoting a culture of health and wholeness. This is an area I plan to explore in greater depth in an upcoming book on the redox health paradigm and its broader ramifications and on the redoxhealth.org website.

Thinking Ahead

The best way to predict the future is to invent it.
—Alan Kay

One of the hazards of writing a health book about cutting-edge research is that the cutting edge keeps moving. You're never done, and your book is outdated when you finish the writing/revision process. At the same time, I've spent a lifetime predicting the future by understanding the ramifications of present realities and trends. I can tell you with some confidence that this book covers or alludes to a broad range of megatrends that will influence the next decade of health research, policy, and practice. My confidence comes not from some Nostradamus-like prescience but rather because new ideas and discoveries always take time to reach critical mass. To the extent that this book is focused on today's cutting-edge research and the ideas and discoveries that I expect to be most impactful, I can look five to ten years out and give you a picture of our health future that has at least a shot at coming true. Thus, I conclude with a forecast—megatrends and specific predictions—to get you thinking and hopefully excited about the progress we can make together.

Megatrend #1: The Rise of Redox Health

Whether or not it is ultimately called redox health is immaterial, in the next decade, I expect it to happen along the following lines:
- Oxidative stress/redox imbalance, inflammation, and stress resilience (general susceptibility to disease) will supplant LDL/lipid management (heart disease-specific) as the primary focus of preventive healthcare.
- Systems thinking and concepts from systems biology and network medicine will increasingly influence western medicine practice and protocols and help us realize precision medicine.

- Precision nutrition, nutritional therapeutics, and lifestyle therapeutics (diet/exercise/sleep/stress management) will rise in prominence with specific applications and protocols for cardiometabolic diseases, cancer prevention, mental health, immunomodulation, autoimmune and inflammatory diseases, aging, cognitive decline, and neurodegeneration and other chronic diseases.
- Neutrophil Lymphocyte Ratio (NLR) or some other redox-relevant biomarker will become routinely used to measure and track inflammation, oxidative stress, and stress resilience.
- Polyphenols and other phytonutrients will rise in importance for cancer prevention, stress resilience, anti-aging, and chronic disease prevention. Modified versions of polyphenols will be patented and become pharmaceuticals.
- Polyphenols and other phytonutrients, often from plant waste byproducts, will increasingly be adopted by the food industry and enter the food supply as a strategy for improving the perceived healthfulness of processed and prepared foods. *Note: this is already happening in the animal feed industry.*
- High-end redox therapeutics, gene therapies, epigenetic manipulation, and treatment of system-specific feedforward loops and pro-inflammatory/pro-oxidant states will join and, in some cases, supplant pharmaceuticals and surgery at the mid to high-end of medicine.
- An Asian, African, or South American country will beat the US and Europe in broad adoption of redox health principles at a national level because the economic incentives to do so will trump healthcare and pharmaceutical industry opposition and inertia.
- Possible: An insurance company will cover a range of polyphenols and other nutraceuticals much as they now incentivize the use of generics. This could be a separate policy, much like vision and dental insurance.
- Improved management of redox, nutritional and immune status will result in improved stress resilience and mental health in populations where it is effectively practiced.

Megatrend #2: The Rise of Mobile Health, Continuous Monitoring, Big Data and AI Influence on Medicine

At its most basic, this is just an extrapolation of existing trends in the smartphone/smartwatch trends. We've got multiple $1 trillion+ companies competing in this space for hegemony. Tech companies have historically created an attractive value proposition with early adopters and then expanded that value proposition and lowered the price point to reach ever broader markets. That said, I expect the following to happen:

- The Apple Watch (currently a class II medical device) and other wearables will become increasingly credible medical devices, adding sensors that detect stress levels, blood pressure, blood glucose. Compared to high-end devices, what they lack in accuracy, they will compensate for through continuous monitoring.
- At some point, your employer, your insurance company, or your health system will buy you a smartwatch as an incentive for you to monitor, maintain and improve your health, and it will make economic sense for them to do it.
- Your health data will eventually be automatically shared with your family physician (with your consent). Privacy laws will need to catch up with the new reality that tech companies are gathering massive amounts of personal health data, and with it comes enormous potential for abuse.
- AI-driven automated analysis services will add value to your health data for both you and your doctor, spotting early warning signs based on multiple correlated biomarkers, positive and negative lifestyle trends.
- At some point, your insurance company will pay for full genome sequencing to incentivize the added value of your medical providers having access to the analysis of your full genome. The price of doing this will continue to fall. Large insurers will cut volume purchase agreements to drive the costs down more quickly. *Note: I have already had both consumer-grade and full-genome tests, the latter with lifetime access to analysis services.*

- The price of health testing will continue to fall, making nutritional testing and more sophisticated diagnostic testing practical and economically viable.
- There will be some manifestation of NLR or Systemic Immune Inflammation (SII) index-tracking on your smartphone/smartwatch.
- Implantable and swallowable medical devices will augment the capabilities of wearables for tracking and diagnostics.
- Probable: Zero interface devices—rings and bands—will become a significant new niche in health tracking wearables as capabilities grow.

Megatrend #3: The Rise of Healthspan Over Lifespan as a Health Outcome

Driven by advances in anti-aging and redox biology research, lifespan will continue to increase, with rising concern for quality of life and delaying age-related loss of function—all under the rubric of healthspan. Beyond that, I expect the following to happen:
- The 80s will become the new 70s for an increasing number of people who effectively practice their resilience habits and maintain healthy redox, nutritional and immune status.
- Self-driving cars, Ubers, delivery services, smartwatches, and other technology assists will allow a growing number of elderly to live independently longer. Many will elect to live at home outside of institutional settings until their deaths.
- Nutrition in retirement communities will be recognized as either contributing to or detracting from residents' health.
- Our ability to extend life medically will ultimately lead to increased de-stigmatization and decriminalization of euthanasia, even as we find ways to extend quality of life/healthspan for a growing segment of the population.
- Age-related eye conditions such as cataracts, macular degeneration, retinopathy will significantly decrease in populations where redox, nutritional and immune status

are properly maintained.
- Probable: Gene therapy will reverse hearing and vision loss before 2030.
- Effective management of redox, nutritional, and immune status will generally lower cancer rates, particularly among the elderly. Chemoprevention with plant polyphenols/phytonutrients will accelerate this trend.
- More effective management of subclinical magnesium deficiency and redox status will significantly decrease atrial fibrillation, arrhythmias, and sudden cardiac death as a middle-age and old-age health concern.
- Increasingly effective amino acid therapeutics (taurine, glycine, l-carnosine/beta-alanine, creatine, l-carnitine) and mitochondrial/metabolic therapeutics (CoQ10/Ubiquinol, AMPK activators, NAD+ repletion, etc.) will significantly reduce sarcopenia and frailty in elderly populations.
- Mitochondrial/metabolic therapeutics (CoQ10/Ubiquinol, AMPK activators, magnesium, l-carnitine, NAD+ repletion, polyphenols, sirtuin activators, etc.) along with improved redox status management will significantly reduce or delay heart failure as a health concern in aging populations.
- Improved nutritional, redox, anti-aging, and mitochondrial therapeutics in association with pharmaceutical advances will reverse trends towards increasing incidence of Alzheimer's and other neurological/neurodegenerative and cognitive disorders in populations where redox health principles are effectively practiced.

These megatrends and predictions, in most instances, already have some current manifestation in research labs across the globe. Thus, while unexpected breakthroughs could accelerate progress or regulatory, legal, and commercial setbacks could prevent some from happening or delay their arrival, I believe all of these are within reach. Writing and now publishing this book has been an initial exercise in envisioning a new healthcare future. As the Alan Kay quote at the beginning of the section advises, let us go and invent it—together.

Postscript

Chasing Health: Reflections on the Journey

There were many times during the writing of this book that I was wracked with self-doubt and bemused by the audacity of a former IT professional writing a book about health and disease. Even at my very best, I'm just one more person who doesn't know everything, researching a topic so vast it can't be fully understood. Ever. So I've had to step back and reflect on the process periodically. What am I learning, not just about health and disease but about research, data, knowledge creation, and human scientific endeavor?

The destination matters. As Stephen Covey says, "Management is doing things right. Leadership is doing the right things."

Long before I considered writing this book, I confronted in my daughter's ADHD diagnosis the limits of human knowledge. Doctors could tell me she had ADHD and give her Ritalin to manage it, but they couldn't tell me why she had it, the root causes, or how to cure it. I needed to understand the root causes, which I believed and still believe is the proper goal and destination of health inquiry. In my IT organization, I would tell my employees that if you are headed in the right direction, even if you don't know exactly where it leads, you will encounter and solve the right problems. So in this book, I am simply modeling that philosophy in the healthcare context, heading in the right direction (understanding root causes), and engaging the global community of scientists and patients to help me solve the problems that arise along the way.

In any journey, the best things that happen along the way are invariably unscripted and serendipitous. Writing this book has been no different. I initially went to PubMed with specific research objectives. I always returned with learnings I never anticipated. Over the years, what began as a body of novel facts has evolved into principles, hypotheses, paradigms, and at its best, something resembling wisdom that will shape my future work. I share the insights below, not as absolutes but as an encouragement to anyone else on a similar journey.

We Know Collectively More Than We Know Individually

> *"Groups are only smart when there is a balance between the information that everyone in the group shares and the information that each of the members of the group holds privately. It's the combination of all those pieces of independent information, some of them right, some of the wrong, that keeps the group wise."*
> — James Surowiecki, The Wisdom of Crowds

While the quote is speaking to organizations, this principle can be applied at global scale, thanks to the Internet and resources like PubMed. In the world of computing, I often remind people that whatever problem you are encountering, someone else has invariably already had it too. Most likely, they have solved it, and you can Google for it. In health research, individual researchers know their specific niche in incredible detail. Still, they can't always know how their work relates to other scientists' work in other fields or what all the ramifications of their work might be. At a minimum, it's difficult for them to explain it to us. So my strategy has been to mine the knowledge of individuals and teams, make connections between bodies of research, and interpret them in understandable, useful, and actionable ways. I find that often the questions I'm asking have already had significant research into them.

Error Happens—We Need to Be Able to Deal with It

> *"There must be no barriers to freedom of inquiry. There is no place for dogma in science. The scientist is free, and must be free to ask any question, to doubt any assertion, to seek for any evidence, to correct any errors."*
>
> — *J. Robert Oppenheimer*

Doctors' deep fear is that their patients will "research" their illness on the Internet and come up with wacko ideas that are at best useless and at worst dangerous. The deep suspicion of patients is that their doctors are not keeping up with the latest research. Both concerns have some basis in reality. As I have researched this book, I have had to acknowledge my own limitations—I am occasionally prone to selection bias. I have an imperfect understanding of the research I'm reading. I also acknowledge the limitations of scientists and their research. Some of the studies are poorly designed, some of the details are wrong, some of the conclusions are speculative or overstated, some of the results are in direct conflict with other studies, some of the writing and spelling is bad, some of the studies are bought and paid for (e.g., food and beverage industry-funded nutritional research), and some of the methodologies are questionable. Anyone who does research needs to evaluate the information they find and make judgments about what to keep and what to discard based on relevance, accuracy, completeness, authoritativeness, bias, conflict of interest, etc. The reader is ultimately the arbiter of whether my judgments are sound.

Spotting Trends in PubMed

"Trends, like horses, are easier to ride in the direction they are going."
— John Naisbitt

In the 1980s, a popular book by John Naisbitt titled *Megatrends* attempted to spot trends using newspapers as closed systems. By watching what new topics entered the paper and what old topics were displaced, Naisbitt could spot societal trends with an impressive degree of accuracy. I've used this technique in my IT career with good success, and now in health research, I found my closed system of choice in PubMed. PubMed is a global database of health research. Its articles are keyword searchable, and the results provide title, abstract, often full text, date of publication, journal, authors, etc. This provides you with a good overview of what is being studied, how intensely it is being studied, whether the research is mature, whether multiple branches of research are studying a particular phenomenon, whether your hypothesis is already being researched, proven, or disproven.

While the average consumer cannot access every article's full text, if possible, read or at least skim the ones available. Not every research article is worthy of being read like a novel, but the best ones are not just really good reads; they are mind-blowing, paradigm-changing works that deserve a much wider audience than they typically get. Also, by engaging the details, you begin to learn what you know and don't know, what's important and what's peripheral, and where the boundaries of knowledge lie for that area of research.

Your First Model Will Be Too Simple

"Everything should be made as simple as possible, but not simpler."
—Albert Einstein

The beauty of this Einstein quote is how it wryly points out that in our desire to simplify we can cross over into simply being wrong. In choosing to focus this book on redox imbalance and the centrality of oxidative and reductive stress in health and disease, I knew there was a risk that the thesis, while deliciously elegant, could be oversimplified to the point of being wrong. After what has become years and thousands of hours of research, I can say with some confidence that the centrality of oxidative/reductive stress and redox imbalance in health and disease has actually held up surprisingly well.

Scientists who believed that antioxidants were a silver bullet for stopping disease have had to temper their enthusiasm and modulate their theories, which is how the paradigm refinement process works. Oxidants play a key signaling role in immune function, signaling, respiration and systemic regulation. Thus far, the greatest challenge has come from mitohormesis researchers, who claim that oxidative stress extends lifespan (think exercise and calorie restriction) by modulating mitochondrial function in ways that make them more resistant to stress. Further, they assert that antioxidants, to the extent that they block mitohormesis, are useless or even dangerous. If this were absolutely true, you wouldn't see health benefits from a phytonutrient-rich, plant-based diet, and you wouldn't see negative health ramifications from starvation and over-exercise. Nevertheless, the research is interesting, and the learnings are being incorporated into a richer, more complex, more accurate model of redox health and disease.

You Will Eventually Break the Old Paradigm

"You believe today's paradigms are not going to change....Ask the caveman then if his paradigms changed or not. Think for yourself you lose. Think for coming generations you win."

— Sameh Elsayed

Along the way, there have been many discoveries that confirmed that I was dealing with a fundamentally different health paradigm—a different way of thinking about health and disease from that of Western medicine as currently practiced. These include

Redox Recycling

The idea that our bodies have systems devoted to recycling and balancing key antioxidants (e.g., glutathione, NADPH, thioredoxin, vitamin C), and key oxidants (NAD+) is revolutionary. It lays the foundation for the concept of stress resilience and antioxidant capacity. We don't just get antioxidants from our food. We generate, store and recycle them in our bodies to maintain health and to be resilient in the face of life's stressors. Our ability to maintain and replenish these redox pools and associated enzymes is intimately linked to our understanding of good health.

Redox Signaling and Epigenetics

Up until the late 1990s, reactive oxygen and nitrogen species (ROS/RNS) were understood entirely in terms of their ability to oxidize and thus damage other molecules. The discovery of the signaling function of these ROS/RNS and their ability to control gene expression evolved alongside the field of epigenetics, which explored the idea that while our genes are fixed, genetic expression is dynamic. Together, redox signaling and epigenetics provided both machinery and processes for understanding health as a dynamic and adaptive process. Redox signaling alerts us to the need to adapt, while epigenetics provides the ability to adapt. On the downside, these same mechanisms can become pathological when the stressors become too high or last too long. The result is disease.

The Curative Power of Plants

In 1979, when Nathan Pritikin published *The Pritikin Program for Diet and Exercise*, the idea that plants could reverse disease was radical. Through the work of people such as Dean Ornish, Caldwell Esselstyn, T. Colin Campbell, John McDougall, Joel Fuhrman, and others, whole food, plant-based diets as potent medical interventions have become firmly and scientifically established. In the last two decades, researchers have leveraged this development to deepen our understanding of both why plants are curative and how the body and disease work. The result has been an explosion of knowledge about plant polyphenols and biochemical pathways such as NRF2, AMPK, FOXO, PGC1a, NF-κB, mTOR, MAPK, ERK, and JNK and their role in health and disease.

The Centrality of Nutrition

A 2016 study reported that med schools provided, on average, 19.6 hours of instruction on nutrition across a four-year curriculum. Less than half of the schools offered a dedicated course in nutrition. This contrasts with the accumulating body of evidence that nutrition provides the biochemical raw materials necessary for health and resilience, that malnutrition is an integral component of disease, and that stress of all kinds degrades nutritional status. In a redox health paradigm, nutrition is at the center because to do otherwise is scientifically indefensible.

Mitohormesis, NAD+, and Reductive Stress

In recent decades, scientists discovered that they could raise glutathione levels with the amino acid N-acetylcysteine (NAC). Given the increasing understanding of glutathione's role in cellular health, NAC seemed destined for wonder-drug status. But then the researchers noticed something odd. Supplementation with NAC blunted the *benefits* of exercising! This research highlighted the importance of low levels of ROS signaling for adaptation to exercise and strengthened the case for the concept of hormesis or mitohormesis—beneficial effects from low levels of oxidative stress. More recently, the discovery of the regulatory function of NAD+ in metabolism and mitochondrial function established the central role of an oxidant (NAD+) in maintaining healthy energy production and an object lesson on how reductive stress could dysregulate a core system (metabolism) underlying health and disease.

The Importance of the Gut Microbiome and Barrier Function

It is hard to fathom that the Western medical paradigm still operates with protocols that treat the GI tract as little more than dumb plumbing. I could easily have written an entire book on the microbiome and its key roles in signaling, regulation of other organ systems, immune health, and barrier maintenance. A healthy gut microbiome is critical for maintaining the gut barrier. Similarly, the same underlying mechanisms that prevent intestinal permeability also keep the vascular barrier healthy. Oxidative stress causes barrier permeability and is caused by barrier permeability and the resulting immune system activation by lipopolysaccharide and other bacterial components.

The Health Implications of a Chronically Activated Immune System

Redox signaling is a logical mechanism for immune system activation since ROS imply both damage to clean up and/or pathogens to fight. Thus, chronically elevated ROS will lead to a chronically-activated immune system. The result is inflammation, downward pressure on immunonutrients, immunoincompetence and/or immune hypersensitivity, and ultimately immunosenescence—the aging and increasingly ineffective immune system.

The Health Implications of a Chronically Activated HPA Axis, Sympathetic Nervous System (SNS), and Renin–Angiotensin–Aldosterone System

Early in the stress response, the HPA axis activates the sympathetic nervous system—your fight or flight system. Oxidative stress keeps the HPA axis, sympathetic nervous system, and the renin-angiotensin-aldosterone system activated. This may sound basic, but the seeds of redox imbalance and downstream dysregulations are sown here, including

- Elevated resting heart rate
- Low heart rate variability (HRV)
- Activated microglial cells/neuroimmune activation and neuroinflammation
- Magnesium efflux leading to intracellular magnesium deficiency
- Dysregulated calcium/magnesium ratio and elevated cellular calcium
- Elevated angiotensin II
- Hyperaldosteronism (and more oxidative stress)
- Increased sodium retention
- Elevated blood pressure
- Elevated fluid retention
- Increased arterial stiffness

The Tight Linkage between Redox Status and Protein Production

Cells have varied functions to carry out, and they rely on a supply of the correct proteins to do so. Oxidative stress causes endoplasmic reticulum (ER) stress and damage to protein production (e.g., unfolded and misfolded proteins). Unchecked, this can result in programmed cell death. In addition to its role in maintaining healthy redox status and immune system functions, Glutathione also helps keep the ER protein factories humming.

We Are Standing on the Shoulders of Giants

> *"But by far the greatest obstacle to the progress of science and to the undertaking of new tasks and provinces therein is found in this—that men despair and think things impossible."*
> — *Sir Francis Bacon*

I am continually amazed by what the global research community has discovered and continues to learn about the workings of health, disease, and, more broadly, life. The emerging picture is more complex, more awe-inspiring, more vast and limitless than we could ever have imagined. Just as early astronomers looked at the sky and saw something incomprehensibly vast, we now peer into a microscope, see microRNA, and must admit that we have barely begun our exploration. This understanding brings both humility that our understanding of health and disease will always be imperfect and the knowledge that our current paradigm is ephemeral and must give way to something better, cheaper, more effective, more aligned with society's goals and aspirations. I'm making a case for redox health as the successor paradigm, but the decision will not be mine.

A Note to Skeptics, Critics, and Detractors

There will invariably be people who find this book and the ideas in it threatening, offensive, presumptuous, even dangerous. Others will simply be skeptical that a body of research resides outside of the current medical paradigm that actually represents an alternative and better paradigm. I would be surprised if it were otherwise, and I welcome constructive criticism and debate. Democrats and Republicans remind us daily that people can look at the same body of information and reach quite different conclusions about how to respond to it.

I have no illusions that this book is perfect. My pedigree for delivering this information is atypical. But to use a metaphor, the global scientific community is holding up a big flashing sign with an arrow that says, "Go this way," and to the extent that we aren't heading that way, I'm simply calling everyone's attention to it.

My commitment to anyone reading this book is that I will continue to listen and synthesize new primary research. The redox health paradigm will continue to evolve and improve as the underlying science advances.

What's Next?

This book represents the first and foundational work in an ecosystem of books that view health, disease, healthcare, and health policy through the lens of a redox health paradigm. As a new paradigm, there are unlimited opportunities for rethinking diseases, care delivery, institutions, industries, and societal problems through the lens of redox health. Example topics might include

- Redox health for patients
- Redox health cooking
- Redox health workouts
- Redox health in K–12 education
- Redox health in college
- Redox health and mental illness
- Redox health in the penal system
- Redox health in the developing world
- Redox health as a path to universal healthcare
- Redox health and healthcare cost control
- Redox health and racial/economic/environmental justice
- Redox health and COVID-19
- Redox health and <insert disease name here>

If you'd like to team up to write one of these books, drop me an email at info@redoxhealth.org, and we can discuss the possibilities.

Beyond books, my fondest hope is that you and a million other scientists, patients, healthcare professionals, and citizen scientists worldwide would join me in crowdsourcing a better, less costly, more effective future of healthcare and health maintenance. If you're interested, drop me an email at info@redoxhealth.org and tell me how you'd like to help. Also, visit https://redoxhealth.org for the latest updates on redox health, along with more in-depth coverage of specific diseases and therapies. A better healthcare future starts now.

Best wishes,

Michael Sherer

> *"Dream no small dreams, for they have no power to move our hearts."*
>
> *—Johann Wolfgang von Goethe.*

Appendix A: Redox Glossary

Adaptive immune system[198] — The adaptive immune system is a subsystem of the human immune system that learns to destroy specific pathogens and remembers them to improve future efficacy. The adaptive immune response is characterized by white blood cell involvement (lymphocytes), with B cells handling antibody responses and T cells handling cell-mediated responses.

Advanced glycation end-products / AGEs[199] — Oxidative stress leads to the increased production of advanced glycation end products (AGEs), proteins, or lipids that become glycated due to exposure to sugars. Sources of AGEs include high-temperature food processing and preparation, and endogenous (internal) production caused by high dietary sugar intake, particularly from high fructose corn syrup. AGEs are toxic and have been shown to cause oxidative stress, mitochondrial dysfunction, insulin resistance, fibrosis, impairment of the transcriptional activity of the nuclear factor erythroid 2-related factor 2 (NRF2), and organ damage.

Aldose reductase[200] — Aldose reductase is an enzyme primarily known for catalyzing glucose reduction to sorbitol, the first step in the polyol pathway of glucose

---

[198] Age-related Oxidative Stress Compromises Endosomal Proteostasis

[199] Dietary Sugars and Endogenous Formation of Advanced Glycation Endproducts: Emerging Mechanisms of Disease

[200] Aldose reductase deficiency leads to oxidative stress-induced dopaminergic neuronal loss and autophagic abnormality in an animal model of Parkinson's disease.

metabolism. Aldose reductase is also involved in dopamine synthesis. The reduction of aldose reductase has been linked to the downregulation of antioxidant enzymes, leading to increased oxidative stress.

Alpha lipoic acid[201] — Alpha lipoic acid (ALA) is the reduced form of lipoic acid. ALA is a naturally occurring thiol antioxidant and glutathione precursor, and it also participates in the recycling of other antioxidants such as vitamin C and vitamin E.

AMPK[202] — AMPK is a key redox and metabolic pathway, protecting cells from oxidative stress as it elevates intracellular NAD+, upregulates sirtuin production, prevents cellular senescence, and promotes autophagy. Recent evidence indicates that AMPK can also upregulate the NRF2 pathway.

Antioxidant capacity/Oxygen radical absorbance capacity (ORAC) is an assay test used to quantify the antioxidant capacity in foods. The USDA maintained a database of ORAC scores for over 300 foods on the premise that foods with high ORAC scores are health-inducing.

Antioxidant response element (ARE) is a genetic sequence found on several genes responsible for detoxification enzymes and cytoprotective proteins. NRF2 binds to ARE in the process of upregulating genes related to cellular defense.

Advanced oxidative protein products (AOPPs) — AOPPs are considered potential biomarkers for oxidative stress. They are oxidized protein byproducts produced during a state of redox imbalance. AOPPs are toxic and pro-inflammatory. They are linked to numerous diseases, including atherosclerosis and kidney disease.

Apoptosis in the cellular lifecycle is programmed cell death. Apoptosis is a controlled process and can be beneficial

---

201 α-Lipoic Acid Ameliorates Oral Mucositis and Oxidative Stress Induced by Methotrexate in Rats. Histological and Immunohistochemical Study

202 AMPK Activation Protects Cells From Oxidative Stress-Induced Senescence via Autophagic Flux Restoration and Intracellular NAD(+) Elevation

to the organism as a part of normal cell turnover, immune function, and protection against pathological dysregulation. However, apoptosis can also become dysregulated and contribute to disease states. Apoptosis contrasts with **necrosis**, which is uncontrolled, damage-driven cell death that is considered uniformly pathological.

Ascorbate — Commonly known as vitamin C, ascorbate is an exogenous antioxidant for humans, meaning there are no internal mechanisms for producing it. Thus, humans get vitamin C from food sources or supplementation. Ascorbate participates in glutathione recycling, and in turn, dehydroascorbic acid, its oxidized form, is recycled to ascorbate by the glutathione system.

Astaxanthin — Astaxanthin is a potent antioxidant found in krill and shellfish. Numerous studies indicate a role for astaxanthin in protecting skin against ultraviolet damage.[203]

Blood-brain barrier/BBB hyperpermeability — The blood-brain barrier (BBB) is a membrane that serves to separate the brain from blood-borne pathogens and the immune system. BBB hyperpermeability is a suspected pathology in neurodegenerative disease, allowing both pathogens and immune system components to come in contact the brain, resulting in increased inflammation and oxidative stress.

Calcium/calcium loading — Cellular calcium dysregulation is an early impact of oxidative stress due to magnesium efflux from the cell. Magnesium is a natural calcium channel blocker, and stress-driven reductions in intracellular magnesium lead to increased intracellular calcium.[204]

Calcium channels — A calcium channel is an ion channel that facilitates calcium movement in and out of the cell.

---

[203] Ng, Qin Xiang et al. "Effects of Astaxanthin Supplementation on Skin Health: A Systematic Review of Clinical Studies." *Journal of dietary supplements*, 1-14. 23 Mar. 2020, doi:10.1080/19390211.2020.1739187

[204] Yasmin, Farzana et al. "Immobilization-induced increases of systolic blood pressure and dysregulation of electrolyte balance in ethanol-treated rats." *Pakistan journal of pharmaceutical sciences* vol. 28,4 (2015): 1365-72.

Carvacrol is a monoterpenoid phenol found in oregano, thyme, and other plants. Carvacrol is a potent antimicrobial agent with antibacterial, antiviral, and antifungal effects.

Catalase is a key antioxidant enzyme that catalyzes the decomposition of hydrogen peroxide into water and oxygen.

Complement system/immune complement system — The **complement system** is a part of the immune system that enhances (complements) the ability of antibodies and phagocytic cells to clear microbes and damaged cells from an organism, promotes inflammation, and attacks the pathogen's plasma membrane.

CoQ/CoQ10/ubiquinol — **Ubiquinol** is an electron-rich (reduced) form of coenzyme Q_{10}. It is an antioxidant molecule involved in energy transfer. The highest concentrations of CoQ10 in tissue of the heart, muscles, liver and kidney. Levels fall with age and correspond with lower energy production.

Curcumin is the principal curcuminoid found in turmeric (*Curcuma longa*). Curcumin is a potent anti-inflammatory with anticancer and antioxidant properties through AMPK and NRF2 activation.

Damage-associated molecular patterns (DAMPs) are components of the innate immune system that can initiate and perpetuate a sterile inflammatory response. In contrast, pathogen-associated molecular patterns (PAMPs) initiate and perpetuate the *infectious* pathogen-induced inflammatory response.

DNA damage is an alteration in the chemical structure of DNA, such as a break in a strand of DNA, a base missing from the backbone of DNA, or a chemically changed base. Redox imbalance can cause DNA damage through oxidation. DNA damage repair via PARP contributes to NAD+ depletion and resulting metabolic dysregulation.

Electron transport — The **electron transport chain (ETC)** is a series of complexes (I through IV) that transfer electrons from electron donors to electron acceptors via redox (both reduction and oxidation occurring simultaneously) reactions. NAD+ supports the efficient operation of the ETC.

Endoplasmic reticulum — The **endoplasmic reticulum (ER)** is a cellular organelle responsible for manufacturing the proteins needed by the cell for proper function. ER stress results in misfolded proteins and activates the unfolded protein response (UPR).

Endotoxin/lipopolysaccharide — **Lipopolysaccharides (LPS)**, also known as **endotoxins**, are large molecules consisting of a lipid and a polysaccharide. LPS is found in the outer membrane of gram-negative bacteria and elicits strong immune responses in animals and humans. Increased gut and vascular permeability allow LPS to pass from the intestine to the bloodstream and are linked to elevated oxidative stress and systemic inflammation.

Endothelial hyperpermeability or **vascular permeability** refers to the state endothelial tight junctions are relaxed, allowing larger molecules to pass through the vessel wall. This is useful for delivering immune components to cells beyond the reach of the vasculature but can also contribute to edema.

Eustress — Beneficial stress—either psychological, physical (e.g., exercise), or biochemical/radiological.

Feedforward loops in biology are concepts borrowed from systems theory describing an element or pathway within a control system that passes a controlling signal without a regulating feedback mechanism. An example of this in the human body would be insulin release based on the presence of glucose in the intestine. The release occurs in anticipation of that glucose being absorbed into the bloodstream.

Flavonoids are a class of plant and fungal polyphenols generally regarded as health-inducing via NRF2 activation. Catechins, quercetin, and rutin are examples of flavonoids.

Gene activation/deactivation — Epigenetic modification of a gene state.

Regulation of gene expression includes a wide range of mechanisms used by cells to increase or decrease the production of specific gene products (protein or RNA).

Glutathione (GSH) is your body's primary endogenous antioxidant, playing a key role in maintaining redox homeostasis. The glutathione system recycles oxidized glutathione (GSSG) to its reduced form (GSH). This system relies on compounds that include precursors (glutamine, cysteine, glycine) and cofactors (vitamin C, vitamin E, vitamins B1, B2, B6, B12, and folate (B9), selenium, magnesium and zinc, and alpha lipoic acid) Glutathione also plays important roles in immune function, protein synthesis, and detoxification.

Glutathione peroxidase is an enzyme family whose main biological role is to protect the organism from oxidative damage. The biochemical function of glutathione peroxidase is to reduce lipid hydroperoxides to their corresponding alcohols and to reduce free hydrogen peroxide to water.

Glutathione reductase or **glutathione-disulfide reductase (GSR)** is an enzyme that in humans is encoded by the GSR gene.

GSSG is the disulfide or oxidized form of glutathione. In living cells, glutathione disulfide is reduced into two molecules of glutathione (GSH) with reducing equivalents from the coenzyme NADPH.

Gut–vascular barrier — First identified in 2015, the gut–vascular barrier performs an analogous function to the blood-brain barrier, which separates the brain from pathogens and the immune system. A dysregulated gut–vascular barrier will allow larger molecules and even bacteria to pass from the intestine into the bloodstream.

Heavy metal toxicity — Heavy metals such as mercury and cobalt are potent oxidative stressors. They are not easily broken down and removed from the system, making them a significant contributor to oxidative stress burden. Chelation, a process that binds and removes metals, is performed by glutathione, alpha lipoic acid, and amino acids such as dimercaptosuccinic acid (DMSA).

Heat shock proteins — HSPs are a family of proteins produced as a part of the cellular stress response. While initially discovered as a response to heat, more recent research indicates that they are produced under numerous stress conditions, including cold and UV light. HSPs are generally considered to be protective and exhibit some overlapping functions with the unfolded protein response.

Heme oxygenase (HO) — Heme oxygenase is an enzyme produced by the heme oxygenase-1 gene regulated by NRF2. HO plays a key role in preventing vascular inflammation, the underlying mechanism of atherosclerosis.

Histamine is a neurotransmitter and signaling molecule produced by mast cells as a response to allergens and pathogens. Histamine and histamine receptors are implicated in several allergic diseases and are responsible for the characteristic symptoms—sneezing, runny nose, watery eyes, and airway inflammation. The polyphenol quercetin is a natural antihistamine and mast cell inhibitor.

Homeostasis refers to the body's capacity to maintain a stable state despite a changing and unpredictable environment. Redox signaling and regulation are important mechanisms in both homeostasis and the associated adaptations to environmental stressors.

HPA axis — The **hypothalamic–pituitary–adrenal axis** (HPA axis) describes a complex set of hormonal and feedback interactions among three endocrine glands: the hypothalamus, the pituitary gland (a pea-shaped structure located below the thalamus), and the adrenal glands (small, conical organs on top of the kidneys). Functionally, the HPA axis is associated with the stress response. Chronic activation and dysregulation of the HPA axis contribute to redox imbalance and dysregulation of the autonomic nervous system, renin-angiotensin-aldosterone system and immune system, metabolic syndrome, and central obesity.

Hydrogen peroxide (H_2O_2) is the most prominent redox signaling molecule due to its stability and ubiquity. H_2O_2

is formed via the detoxification of superoxide molecules by superoxide dismutase. Dysregulated energy metabolism leads to the overproduction of superoxide radicals and elevated levels of H_2O_2, the central features of oxidative stress and redox imbalance.

Hydroxyl radical — The **hydroxyl radical**, ·OH, is a highly reactive and short-lived molecule formed when hydrogen peroxide interacts with Fe2 via a Fenton reaction. Hydroxyl radicals are primary actors in DNA damage and cellular membrane damage. Plant polyphenols are notable scavengers of hydroxyl radicals.

Hyperaldosteronism, also **aldosteronism**, is a pathological state where elevated levels of aldosterone hormone in the blood lead to urinary magnesium and calcium loss, hyperparathyroidism, oxidative stress, and intracellular calcium loading, key mechanisms in the pathogenesis and progression of cardiometabolic diseases.

Hyperparathyroidism is an increase in parathyroid hormone (PTH) levels in the blood. Parathyroid hormone regulates serum calcium levels. Thus, the condition is linked to aldosteronism as the body attempts to offset urinary calcium loss.

Immune system activation occurs in response to pathogenic invasion or physical damage, or trauma. Redox signaling from these stressors activates the NF-κB pathway, which initiates and regulates the immune response.

Inflammation is part of the complex biological response of body tissues to harmful stimuli, such as pathogens, damaged cells, or irritants. It is a protective response involving immune cells, blood vessels, and molecular mediators.

Inflammatory cascade — Inflammation is typically triggered by a toxic or pathogenic insult followed by oxidative stress, NF-κB activation, TNF-alpha and IL-1B production, and a cascade of additional inflammatory cytokines, hence the phrase "inflammatory cascade." This concept overlaps with the idea of feedforward loops and pro-oxidant states.

Innate immune system is an important subsystem of the overall immune system that comprises the cells and mechanisms that defend the host from infection by other organisms. This includes the epithelium and endothelium, involving virtually every surface area where the body could come in contact with its environment.

Intestinal permeability — Under normal circumstances, the intestinal wall exhibits some degree of permeability, which allows nutrients to pass through the gut, while also maintaining a barrier function to keep potentially harmful substances from leaving the intestine and migrating to the body more widely. Gut dysbiosis and oxidative stress can cause increased intestinal permeability, leading to systemic inflammation and oxidative stress and, in extreme circumstances, sepsis.

Iron is a necessary nutrient that needs to be maintained in balance. Low iron (anemia) is associated with fatigue and other symptoms, including rapid heart rate, shortness of breath, pale skin, and cold hands and feet, while oxidative stress and mitochondrial dysfunction are associated with low and high iron levels.

Lactoferrin (LF) is an iron-binding antimicrobial peptide that is part of the innate immune system. LF is found in most bodily fluids and in particularly high levels in mammalian breast milk. Lactoferrin exerts antifungal, antiviral, and antibacterial effects in those fluids and can bind and sequester lipopolysaccharide in the blood.

Lectins are carbohydrate-binding proteins found in plants and animals. Plant sources of lectins include beans, grains, and nightshade vegetables. Wheat gluten is perhaps the most well-known lectin. Health concerns surrounding lectins are primarily centered on the potential for damage to the intestinal lining and intestinal permeability, a source of chronic inflammation and oxidative stress.

Lectin complement pathway is one of three pathways that can activate the immune complement system, a part of the innate immune system. Inappropriate or dysregulated activation of the immune complement system can result in damage to host tissue and cells.

Leukocytes — White blood cells. There are several types of leukocytes, including lymphocytes, granulocytes, monocytes, and macrophages.

Magnesium/magnesium efflux — **Magnesium** is an essential element **in biological systems,** present in every cell. Magnesium occurs typically as the Mg^{2+} ion and is considered an antioxidant mineral. Among its many roles, magnesium is a glutathione cofactor necessary for maintaining healthy redox status. Magnesium is depleted by catecholamines (stress hormones) and expelled from the cell into the serum due to psychological stress. Low magnesium levels are implicated in every pathology of heart disease and are critical for the heart's proper electrical function.

Mast cell — A type of white blood cell that is a part of the immune and neuroimmune systems. Mast cell activation results in the release of histamine and heparin. Along with eosinophils and basophils, mast cells play a central role in allergic conditions.

Metabolic endotoxemia — Increased intestinal or gut–vascular permeability allows lipopolysaccharide (aka endotoxin) to pass from the gut lumen into the bloodstream, causing a condition called metabolic endotoxemia. Elevated levels of LPS in the bloodstream are associated with most inflammatory diseases, including diabetes, depression, anxiety, psychosis, osteoporosis, liver disease, etc.

Mitochondrial biogenesis is the process by which cells increase their individual mitochondrial mass and number to increase the production of ATP. Mitochondria biogenesis is regulated by AMPK and promoted by sirtuins (SIRT1). Exercise is one of the most effective means of promoting mitochondrial biogenesis.

Mitochondrial dysfunction — An early impact of oxidative stress, mitochondrial dysfunction can result from loss of antioxidant capacity, depletion of NAD+, and associated dysregulation of the electron transport chain. The result is fewer, smaller, and less healthy mitochondria lowered energy production and increased mitochondrial ROS production due to decreased efficiency in the electron transport chain.

mTor pathway — The **mechanistic target of rapamycin (mTOR)** is a kinase that in humans is encoded by the *MTOR* gene. mTOR signaling is involved in regulation of growth and metabolism. mTOR activation is implicated in numerous diseases, including cancer, diabetes, neurodegeneration, epilepsy, lupus, etc.

N-acetylcysteine (NAC) is a first-line therapy used to treat acetaminophen overdose and to loosen thick mucus in cystic fibrosis or chronic obstructive pulmonary disease. NAC is a source of cysteine and has been experimentally shown to raise glutathione levels in humans. NAC is also a potent antimicrobial agent that shortens the duration and severity of respiratory infections by breaking down bacterial biofilms.

NAD+ is a major redox metabolite found in all living cells. NAD+ plays an important regulatory role in metabolism and is a substrate for sirtuin production and the DNA repair enzyme PARP. NAD+ repletion is an emerging therapeutic strategy for anti-aging and metabolic dysregulation.

NAD/NADH — The NAD redox couple includes NAD+ (the oxidized form) and NADH (the reduced from). NAD+ is notable for regulating metabolism and raw material for sirtuin production and DNA repair (PARP).

NADP/NADPH — The NADP redox couple includes NADP (the oxidized form) and NADPH (the reduced form). For redox health, the NADP pool needs to be maintained in a reduced state. A higher NADP/NADPH ratio will result in the overproduction of reactive species.

Necrosis refers to premature cell death from cell injury. Unlike **apoptosis**, necrosis is uncontrolled and uniformly associated with pathology.

NF-κB (nuclear factor kappa-light-chain-enhancer of activated B cells) is a protein complex that controls transcription of DNA, cytokine production, and cell survival. NF-κB both initiates and regulates the immune response and is activated by redox signaling.

Nitric oxide (NO) is a free radical and has important signaling functions in the vascular system. Under oxidative stress, superoxide binds with NO to form peroxynitrite, a toxic compound that increases oxidative stress and reduces NO availability in the vasculature.

NRF2 — Nuclear factor (erythroid-derived 2)-like 2 is a transcription factor that in humans is encoded by the NFE2L2 gene. Activation of the NRF2 pathway exerts epigenetic control of over 200 genes associated with cellular defense. NRF2 activation is generally viewed as health-inducing and a core benefit of exercise, plant-based diets, fasting, and other eustressors.

Osteoblasts are cells tasked with synthesizing bone. Oxidative stress can inhibit osteoblast formation, resulting in bone loss.

Osteoclast is a type of bone cell that breaks down bone tissue. This function is critical in the maintenance, repair, and remodeling of bone. Oxidative stress can induce osteoclast formation and an osteoclast/osteoblast imbalance that results in bone pathologies such as osteoporosis.

Oxidative damage — Reactive oxygen and nitrogen species cause oxidative damage to a variety of molecules, including proteins, carbohydrates, fats, and DNA. These oxidized molecules can be useful biomarkers for measuring levels of oxidative stress.

Oxidative phosphorylation is the metabolic pathway in which cells use enzymes to oxidize nutrients, thereby releasing energy used to reform ATP.

Oxidative stress reflects an imbalance between reactive oxygen species and the body's capacity to detoxify or reduce those reactive species or repair the resulting damage. Along with reductive stress, oxidative stress is a manifestation of redox imbalance.

Pathogen-associated molecular patterns, or **PAMPs**, are molecules associated with groups of pathogens recognized by cells of the innate immune system.

Parasympathetic nervous system is one of the three divisions of the autonomic nervous system, the others being the sympathetic nervous system and enteric nervous system. It is referred to as the "rest and repair" or "feed and breed" system in popular parlance.

Parathyroid hormone is a hormone secreted by the parathyroid glands. Parathyroid regulates serum calcium and is important in bone remodeling, an ongoing process in which bone tissue is alternately resorbed and rebuilt over time.

PARP is a family of proteins involved in several cellular processes such as DNA repair, genomic stability, and programmed cell death. NAD+ is consumed in PARP production, and thus oxidative stress-driven DNA damage indirectly leads to NAD+ depletion and mitochondrial dysfunction.

Pathological signaling is contrasted with physiological or normal signaling. Physiological redox signaling is generally understood in terms of serum H_2O_2 levels ≤ 10 nM and pathological signaling being > 100 nM.[205]

Peroxynitrite is a reactive nitrogen species (RNS) with the formula $ONOO^-$. Peroxynitrite is formed when superoxide ($O_2 \cdot$) molecules react with nitric oxide (NO). Peroxynitrite is both toxic and reduces NO availability in the vascular system.

Polyphenols are a class of phytonutrients characterized by the presence of large multiples of phenol structural units. Polyphenols are low-level oxidative stressors with hormetic effects through NRF2 stimulation.

Precursor — A chemical compound that is transformed into another compound via a chemical reaction as a part

---

[205] Sies, Helmut. "Hydrogen peroxide as a central redox signaling molecule in physiological oxidative stress: Oxidative eustress." *Redox biology* vol. 11 (2017): 613-619. doi:10.1016/j.redox.2016.12.035

of a biochemical pathway is a precursor. For example, cysteine is a glutathione precursor, along with glycine and L-glutamine.

Protein folding is the physical process by which a protein chain acquires its native three-dimensional structure, which takes place in the endoplasmic reticulum. Protein folding can be disrupted by oxidative stress and associated endoplasmic reticulum stress.

Proteome — The proteome refers to the complete set of proteins expressed by an organism or specific cell type. The term is a blend of *proteins* and *genome*. Proteomics is the study of the proteome.

Pterostilbene is a stilbenoid polyphenol chemically related to resveratrol. Pterostilbene is found in blueberries and grapes and is considered a promising therapeutic compound for various cancers, diabetes, heart disease, and neurodegenerative diseases.

Quercetin is a flavonoid polyphenol found in apples, onions, and other plants. Quercetin is a widely-studied compound, referenced in 20,000+ articles on PubMed. Quercetin is an antioxidant, antihyperlipidemic, anti-inflammatory, antitumor, antihistamine, antidiabetic, antinociceptive compound. Most recently, quercetin has received research attention as a potential prophylactic against COVID-19 infection.

Reactive nitrogen species (RNS) are nitrogen-containing oxidants derived from nitric oxide (•NO) and superoxide ($O_2^{\cdot}$). Examples of RNS include nitric oxide (NO), peroxynitrite (ONOO·), and nitrogen dioxide (NO_2). Nitric oxide has important signaling functions in the vasculature, while peroxynitrite plays a pathological role, both as a toxic compound responsible for vascular damage and for reducing NO availability.

Reactive oxygen species (ROS) are reactive chemical species containing oxygen. Examples include hydrogen peroxide, superoxide, hydroxyl radical, and singlet oxygen.

Renin-angiotensin-aldosterone system (RAAS) — The RAAS is activated by the HPA axis as part of the stress response. Catecholamines stimulate increased renin release in the kidneys, leading to increased angiotensin and angiotensin 2 levels, fluid retention, hypertension, arterial stiffness, and increased stroke risk.

Redox imbalance — Generally assumed to be elevated oxidative stress and reduced antioxidant capacity, though it also includes reductive stress, where antioxidants suppress physiological redox signaling.

Redox signaling — In the past two decades, substantial evidence has emerged that ROS are essential second messengers in innate and adaptive immune cells. Yet, increased ROS levels within immune cells can result in hyperactivation of inflammatory responses resulting in tissue damage and pathology.

Reductive stress is the counterpart to **oxidative stress**, where electron acceptors are expected to be mostly reduced. It can be caused by excess amounts of glutathione and can contribute to cytotoxicity.

Resveratrol — Resveratrol is a stilbenoid polyphenol, found in grapes and other plants. Resveratrol has received significant attention from the popular health press as an anti-aging compound and beneficial component of the Mediterranean diet. In research circles, resveratrol is recognized as a calorie restriction mimetic that lengthens lifespan in model organisms.

Rutin — Rutin is a flavonoid polyphenol that is found in asparagus, buckwheat, and other plants. Notable actions of rutin include raising nitric oxide availability in the vasculature and stimulating the production of SIRT1.

Senescence — Aging cells with shortened telomeres and no longer able to divide are said to have reached a senescent state. Senescent cells give off damage-associated molecular patterns (DAMPs) to alert the immune system. An aging immune system eventually fails to remove senescent cells with associated pathology in diseases such as pulmonary fibrosis.

Static ORP (sORP) — A valuable "snapshot" of current redox balance, which appears to correlate with illness, injury severity, and mortality. A higher sORP reading is indicative of oxidative stress.

Superoxide radical. The O_2 radical is typically produced by mitochondria and quickly reduced to H_2O_2 by superoxide dismutase. The resulting H_2O_2 molecules are then further reduced to water and oxygen by catalase.

Superoxide dismutase. One of the body's primary endogenous antioxidant enzymes. Superoxide dismutase reduces the superoxide free radical into $2\ HO_2 \rightarrow O_2 + H_2O_2$.

Sympathetic nervous system activation. Stress and oxidative stress lead to the activation of the sympathetic nervous system, known popularly as the "fight or flight" system. Prolonged or hyperactivation of the sympathetic nervous system is associated with autonomic nervous system disorders, including elevated resting heart rate and hypertension and cardiometabolic disease.

Telomere — Telomeres are protein structures found at the end of DNA strands that protect the DNA from damage during division. Telomere shortening is associated with aging, cellular senescence, and apoptosis. Oxidative stress is a contributing factor to telomere shortening.

Tumor necrosis factor (TNF) is a superfamily of proteins with diverse functions in cell cycle regulation, including survival, proliferation, differentiation, and death. TNF alpha is an inflammatory cytokine upregulated by NF-κB and is associated with immune system activation and regulation.

Transcriptome — The sum total of all the messenger RNA molecules expressed from the genes of an organism.

Unfolded protein response (UPR) is a cellular stress **response** related to endoplasmic reticulum (ER) stress and disrupted protein folding. The UPR is highly conserved in mammalian species, as well as yeast and worms. The UPR optimizes the ER to manage protein folding correctly, and if necessary, initiates apoptosis or autophagy in cells that are irreversibly damaged.

Vascular endothelial growth factor (VEGF) is typically upregulated by oxidative stress and is associated with new vessel growth and tumor formation.

Zinc — An antioxidant metal with diverse roles, including 200 zinc enzymes and over 3,000 zinc proteins. Low zinc status increases oxidative stress in the body and negatively impacts immune status and DNA damage repair

---

Thanks for reading "One Disease: Redox Imbalance."

Don't forget to check out the bonus content on our website:

https://redoxhealth.org/bonus/

About the Author

Michael Sherer, a health researcher and author, is a member of the Society for Redox Biology and Medicine and the American Society for Nutrition. In One Disease: Redox Imbalance, his passion for health, nutrition, technology, and cutting-edge research are on full display. The result is a book that will change how you think about health, disease, and healthcare.

Throughout his thirty-year career in IT leadership, Michael Sherer has been called a visionary, an interdisciplinary problem solver, a futurist, a systems thinker, and a trendspotter. Family health issues led Sherer to apply these skills to a broad range of medical research. They ultimately spurred him to leave IT for the uncharted waters of cutting-edge medical research and health writing. *One Disease: Redox Imbalance* is a foundational work and the first in a series of books applying the principles of redox health to help people live longer healthier lives, and provide more effective, lower-cost healthcare models for the societies they live in.

Made in the USA
Monee, IL
18 September 2021